The Best Kept Secrets
.to
Healthy Aging

Presented by the
Purity Research Department

Co-Authors Dr. Neil Levin DC

Jason Kam, Dr. Irfan Qureshi ND

Foreword by
Dr. Barry S. Kendler, PhD, FACN, CNS

The Purity Research Department
Co-Authors: Dr. Neil Levin DC, Jason Kam, Dr. Irfan Qureshi ND

Foreword by Dr. Barry S. Kendler, PhD, FACN,CNS

Copyright © 2009 by Purity Research Department

Published by Purity Products
200 Terminal Drive
Plainview, NY 11803

www.purityproducts.com

First Edition, November 2006

Second Edition, September 2009

ISBN 10: 0-9790588-0-5
ISBN 13: 978-0-9790588-0-6

Ordering information: Single copies and quantity discounts are available from the publisher, Purity Products, 200 Terminal Drive, Plainview, NY 11803. Telephone (888) 313-7873, **www.purityproducts.com** or e-mail customerservice@purityproducts.com.

Table of Contents

Foreword

A new era in nutritional science is currently emerging—one that is built on a foundation of **evidence-based nutraceutical use**, strongly supported by scientifically sound and reproducible research and sharply contrasted with dietary supplement use previously based on questionable studies or anecdotal information.

Although the biomedical literature on evidence-based nutraceutical use is vast and steadily increasing, this research has been largely ignored by most mainstream health care professionals, especially conventional medical doctors. One reason for this is that while enormous financial resources from the pharmaceutical industry are targeted for marketing drugs, only a fraction of this amount is available for publicizing nutraceuticals. However, many health care professionals, including MDs, DOs, DCs, NDs, nutritionists, and nurse practitioners have included nutraceuticals in their practices with very favorable outcomes. That the public is becoming aware of these alternative or complementary health providers is evidenced by huge out-of-pocket expenditures for their services.

Moreover, nutraceutical use directly by the public is increasing steadily as more and more people are becoming aware of their benefits in supporting all facets of health. This has led to burgeoning sales in recent years of omega-3 fatty acids, coenzyme Q-10, phytonutrients, and numerous other products.

Most of the studies supporting nutraceutical use may be accessed on-line without charge by using federal government databases, such as PubMed, and by publications such as this book, which documents the scientific literature supporting evidence-based nutraceutical use. These resources provide consumers with an opportunity to improve their health status, in conjunction with guidance provided by knowledgeable health care providers.

Sincerely,

Barry S. Kendler, PhD, FACN, CNS
Professor of Nutrition
Human Nutrition Institute
University of Bridgeport
Bridgeport, CT

Is Healthy Aging for Real?

Is it possible? Are there choices that we as individuals can make on a daily basis that can support our health and even improve it? Everyone knows the saying "Prevention is better than cure". But not everyone understands what that really means. For years now, we've been bombarded by products touted for their "anti-aging" benefits, only to be disappointed by the science and the results. There's so much background noise out there that it's difficult to distinguish between hype and reality. What really works? What really doesn't? And how do we know?

It's important to realize that there are traditional systems of medicine, such as the ancient Chinese, Ayurvedic (Indian sub-continent) and Unani (Greco-Arabic) traditions that have been in existence for thousands of years, each one of which was designed to be a complete way of life; not just a means to ward off disease, but a means to attain optimal health. Each are based on sound principles that include dietary guidelines, health-promoting lifestyle habits, and nutritional and botanical supplements designed to restore any perceived imbalances that get in the way of achieving health and wellness. Remember now that these systems have been in existence for thousands of years, and they continue to thrive today. That's thousands of years of refreshing and refinement based on what works and what doesn't.

This "experimentation" leads to a strong base on which to establish the fundamental principles of Healthy Aging.

> "Taken together, the ancient wisdom with the modern science allow us to pick and choose from the best of both worlds and establish the keys to aging healthfully."

But we live in the Modern World, a world ruled by science. Science is the "Gold Standard" paradigm through which the effectiveness of all things is to be measured. Thus, if something isn't borne out scientifically (provided it's been studied well, of course), it is to be rejected. This is rightfully so. After all, this is the most objective way there is to measure the effectiveness of various treatments. Thankfully, there exist tens of thousands of scientific papers detailing several aspects of different therapeutics used in traditional methods of medicine. These papers as a whole provide tremendous insight into how the wisdom of ancient healers can benefit our lives given the complexities of the fast-paced world in which we live. Thus, taken together, the ancient wisdom with the modern science allow us to pick and choose from the best of both worlds and establish the keys to aging healthfully - keys that are not hype, but based on sound principles that make logical sense and are supported by scientific investigation. The steps to Healthy Aging are not a mystery. They are a combination of fundamentals including diet, lifestyle choices and supplementation with key nutritional cofactors that lead to vibrant health and support optimal wellness.

Focusing on factors that people themselves are in control of empowers them to take charge of their own wellness. Nature has endowed our bodies with tremendous self-healing capacity. Sometimes it's just a matter of providing the right ingredients to make a successful recipe. The secret is being able to recognize the necessary ingredients and providing them in the right amounts.

This book aims to discuss some of the fundamental choices we all can make that will improve our well-being. It also aims to present the research supporting the use of key nutrients and lifestyle choices that promote health and put forth a strategy that you can begin to implement to optimize the benefits of nature's healing wisdom.

The book is organized into three major sections. The first section features an in-depth discussion of several groundbreaking nutrients or nutrient groups that serve as core ingredients in the recipe for achieving optimal health and wellness.

The second section covers dietary and lifestyle factors, as well as key health-promoting principles covering several organs and systems that lay the groundwork for healthy aging. Nutritional factors that facilitate the achievement of these objectives are also highlighted.

The third section of the book contains guidelines for developing a "Healthy Aging" plan that suits your needs and provides practical guidance on how you can implement the principles discussed in the first two sections of this book into your daily life. The purpose of this book is to give you the tools you need to live an active and prosperous lifestyle that promotes health and wellness. You are ultimately responsible for your own health. So take charge today!

Section I

Super Nutrients for Healthy Aging

1

Your Mother was Right – Fish Is Brain Food

(and Heart Food and Joint Food and Skin Food and Eye Food and....)

Life starts out tough (you can't talk, you can't move, you're surrounded by strangers...) and only gets tougher as you get older. Was it always this way? Maybe...but then again, people used to be satisfied sitting on their porches watching the world go by after age 65. Not anymore – you want to be vibrant and active in all ways. What is the single most important thing you can do to keep the forces of nature at bay?

Of course, you can spend the rest of your life reading the many, many books out there that recommend nutritional means of achieving (they hope) "healthy aging." And then you can spend all of your time downing dietary supplements by the handful as you try to implement all of that advice. But unless you're addressing a very specific concern (such as poor digestion), you really want a simpler answer.

In a word (actually 4), the simple answer is: fish and **fish oils**.

The Oils That Form the Foundation of a Long Healthy Life

Anthropologists (not physicians or nutritionists!) first noticed that even though the Inuit, native people of Greenland, ate huge amounts of fat (from the sea animals and fish they hunted), they seemed to maintain excellent heart health. Investigations by nutrition-minded researchers led to the conclusion that there was something about the nature of all that fat they were eating that was actually protecting the Inuit from the harmful effects that would be expected if the same amount of beef fat was eaten every day.

To summarize decades of research, it turns out that it is the **omega-3 fatty acids** (called "fish oils" because they are mostly found in cold water ocean fish) that are the source of the "heart healthy" effects of eating ocean fish. Virtually every scientific study of these food sources published since the 1970's has revealed yet another health benefit that can be obtained from eating fish from cold-water oceans or by dietary supplementation with their omega-3 oils. Research shows that these nutrients support more than just the heart and cardiovascular system – they can help maintain brain function, help minimize skin reactions to sunlight and other inflammatory triggers and contribute to smooth flexible movement. The avalanche of reliable scientific findings supporting these conclusions provides ample motivation for making cold-water fish and fish oils a fundamental component of your diet.

Fish Oils – What are They?

The two most important fish oils are **eicosapentaenoic acid (EPA)** and **docosahexaenoic acid (DHA)**. These long names reflect their chemical structures; both EPA and DHA (most people use their nicknames) are very long-chain **polyunsaturated fatty acids (PUFA)** commonly found in most cold-water species of ocean fish, especially tuna, salmon and mackerel. The term "omega-3" recognizes the crucial difference in structure that distinguishes them from the "omega-6 PUFA" you are used to getting from vegetable oils.

This difference is so important that the human body cannot efficiently make EPA or DHA from the other fatty acids – the fish oils are dietary essentials that must be consumed from foods or dietary supplements in order for human life to thrive. (A very small amount of EPA may be made from plant-based omega-3 fatty acids, but this process is extremely inefficient, as extra steps are required by the body to perform this conversion.) Although a little EPA can be converted to DHA, obviously it would be much more efficient to consume both preformed EPA and DHA, which are already in forms that can be incorporated into cells. Almost all of the EPA and DHA that is consumed is absorbed and a study published in the journal *Circulation* found that the amounts of EPA and DHA circulating in the blood and being added into your cells and tissues are directly dependent upon how much of each of these fish oils is eaten.[1] When EPA and DHA reach the body's tissues and cells they are incorporated into the structural lipids that make up cell, nuclear and mitochondrial membranes. These membranes absolutely require EPA and DHA in order to function properly - they aid in cell-to-cell communication and facilitate the flow of nutrients into cells as well as the removal of toxins from cells. Improperly incorporated fatty acids (not the preferential ones like EPA and DHA) can hinder these important cellular functions and impair cellular metabolism, leading to unhealthy cells and therefore unhealthy organs. EPA and DHA are thus essential components of every cell in the body.

Fish Oils and a Healthy Heart

Omega-3 essential fatty acids from fish oil have an influence on the entire cardiovascular system; from their impact on how the heart beats to how much pressure your blood puts on your arteries to the health of the heart muscle itself. Proper functionality of every aspect of this system is dependent on these fatty acids in one way or another. We are all aware of the benefits of exercise on cardiovascular health. However, fish oil supplementation may have added benefits above and beyond those of exercise alone. These have been highlighted in a recent study published in the *American Journal of Clinical Nutrition*[2] Researchers looked at the effects of fish oil supplementation in a group of individuals and compared this to a second group consuming fish oil and including regular exercise as a part of their daily regimen. Researchers also looked at a group consuming sunflower oil and exercising regularly, while a fourth group was designated as the control and consumed sunflower oil alone. They found that both fish oil intake and exercise independently contributed to a reduction of body fat. Fish oil also improved several measures of cardiovascular function and enhanced the health of the arteries. This highlights the beneficial effects of fish oil alone and in combination with regular exercise to support healthy cardiovascular function.

> *"Fish oil intake and exercise independently contributed to a reduction of body fat."*

The Rhythm of Your Heart Beating

The contractile rhythms of the heart muscle are produced by synchronized waves of electrical excitation that are communicated through the heart. However, the beat of even a healthy heart is not absolutely regular. The beat varies as the cardiovascular system adjusts to moment-by-moment changes in demand. The ability of the heart to adjust its rhythms is called "heart rate variability" (HRV) and the greater the HRV the better able the heart is to fine tune its beat-to-beat timing without overreacting.

EPA and DHA work together to increase the heart muscle's ability to respond to changing demands. A study published in the *American Journal of Clinical Nutrition* showed that daily dietary supplements of 800 mg of EPA plus 900 mg of DHA for 12 weeks given to a group of healthy men and women with low HRV nearly normalized this important paprameter.[3] The improvements were found to be dose-dependant as greater effects were shown when even more EPA and DHA were consumed. In a separate study 6 months of dietary supplementation with fish oils (2000 mg total every day) increased HRV in elderly men and women nursing home residents.[4]

What is even more interesting is that supplementation with these omega-3 fats doesn't disturb HRV in individuals with normal values. A randomized placebo-controlled clinical trial published in the *American Heart Journal* found that dietary supplementation with EPA (700 mg/day) and DHA (560 mg/day) for 12 weeks had no influence in middle-aged men and women with normal heart rate variability, confirming the safety of fish oil supplements when they are consumed to maintain normal heart function.[5] Further research has demonstrated the superiority of fish oils over olive oil in maintaining cardiac stability.[6] These studies serve to show that EPA and DHA intake has heart function modulating effects, rather than potentiating effects, meaning that omega-3 fatty acids support normalization of heart function in individuals and are not over-stimulating. This effect also points to the safety of long-term use of fish oils for cardiac support as a part of a wellness regimen.

Are Things Going Too Fast?

Healthy cardiovascular function is dependent on the ability of the heart to adjust its pumping rate with different activity levels. This is an important mechanism employed by the body to allow for the efficient circulation of oxygen depending on metabolic needs. At times of rest, the heart rate should be slower and during times of exertion, the rate speeds up to compensate for increased metabolism. Research suggests that fish oil supplementation can normalize resting heart rate by enhancing the heart's ability to pump efficiently. In a 2005 paper, researchers analyzed published research dealing with the effects of fish oil supplementation on human heart rate.[7] The conclusion of this analysis was that fish oil supplementation led to a calming of resting heart rate to normal levels. This beneficial effect allows the body to better compensate for changes in metabolic needs and contributes to overall cardiovascular functionality.

How Wide Open is Your Circulation?

Healthy circulatory function is of paramount importance to optimal health and is an integral component of cardiovascular function. The health of the arteries and veins, as well as their pliability and compliance (their ability to adjust to differences In blood flow), is critical for supporting the optimal function of all organs and systems throughout the body. All of these systems depend on the critical flow of nutrients through the blood to nourish their function. Impaired circulatory function can inhibit this crucial nutrient exchange, leading to less than optimal organ function. One of the most important measures you can take to keep your circulatory system as healthy as possible for as long as possible is to increase your intake of essential EPA and DHA. A growing body of clinical research supports this advice. For example, the results of a study published in the *Annals of Internal Medicine* demonstrated that daily dietary supplementation with 2100 mg of EPA and 1050 mg of DHA promoted healthy circulation in the coronary arteries of men and women.[8] Maintaining smooth circulation enhances the heart's ability to deliver the freshly oxygenated blood your organs and tissues need.

Maintaining Lipid Levels that are Already in the Normal Range?

Maintaining healthy levels of blood lipids, including cholesterol and triglycerides, is important for long-term wellness and plays a major part in the health of the cardiovascular system. We're all aware of the effects of elevated blood lipid levels. However, lipid levels that are too low can also be detrimental to health. A healthy balance of cholesterol and triglycerides is necessary for optimal cardiovascular function. As is evident from the advice given by the National Cholesterol Education Program of the National Institutes of Health, maintaining healthy plasma triglyceride concentration is one vital component in maintaining cardiovascular health. Dietary supplementation with fish oils has been shown in several studies to support plasma triglyceride concentrations that are already in the normal range. For example, a recent study conducted in healthy men found that daily dietary supplementation with 1200 mg of EPA plus 800 mg of DHA for 4 weeks provided invaluable assistance to the body's efforts to maintain healthy plasma triglyceride concentrations.[9] Several other published trials support this ability of fish oil and specifically the fatty acids DHA and EPA.

Eating fatty acids – fish oils – to support healthy levels of fats in the blood – what a concept! This is just one of the reasons that fish oils are so special. This also illustrates the fact that eating fat is not necessarily bad. What's more important is the type of fat one consumes. Consuming healthy fats is an important part of eating for health and healthy aging.

Feeling the Pressure?

Variations in blood pressure levels occur throughout the day in healthy individuals. Blood pressure is a measure of how the cardiovascular system compensates to handle the circulatory demands of the body. It's a mechanism used by the body to ensure adequate flow of nutrients and oxygen to the peripheral organs and tissues. As we age, however, a number of factors can affect the ability of the cardiovascular system to maintain healthy circulation and blood pressure levels. A major factor is the health of the arteries and veins, and their ability to expand and contract with changes in heart rate and circulatory flow. The omega-3 fatty acids EPA and DHA support the health of arteries and veins by maintaining their ability to expand and contract - also known

"Fish oils relax arterial smooth muscle, producing more flexible blood vessels that are better able to adapt to changing demands, which can contribute to the maintenance of already normal, healthy levels of blood pressure."

as compliance. Since these fats are incorporated into the cells that make up the linings of blood vessels, they support the healthy function of these vessels and their compliance. Given this ability, it is not surprising that optimal intake of these fatty acids may promote the maintenance of blood pressure levels already within the normal range. Several studies suggest that EPA and DHA do just that. A study published in the journal *Circulation* showed that dietary supplement-ation with fish oils (2000 mg of EPA plus 1200 mg of DHA) daily for 12 weeks helped otherwise generally healthy men and women maintain blood pressure levels in the normal range.[10]

Further research confirms the mechanism of fish oils that we talked about above - namely that they support the compliance of blood vessels. An article published in the *American Journal of Clinical Nutrition* demonstrated that fish oils relax arterial smooth muscle, producing more flexible blood vessels that are better able to adapt to changing demands[11], which can contribute to the maintenance of already normal, healthy levels of blood pressure.

What do the Experts Say?

The "heart healthy" benefits of fish oils have been shouted from the rooftops. In 2002, the American Heart Association (AHA) concluded that the daily consumption of 500 mg to 1800 mg of EPA + DHA (either as fatty fish or supplements) promoted a healthy heart and cardiovascular system. According to the AHA, daily intakes of 2000 mg to 4000 mg of both EPA and DHA promote healthy plasma triglyceride levels. Further conclusions by the AHA in their 2002 scientific paper include the fact that omega-3 fatty acids support normal heart rhythms and promote healthy blood pressure maintenance. In March of 2004, the U.S. Department of Health and Human Services announced its agreement with the conclusions reached by the AHA.

The Institute of Medicine of the National Academies of Science in its 2005 advisory on macronutrient intakes identified increased heart and cardiovascular health as specific potential health benefits to be derived from increased consumption of cold-water fish and fish oils.[12] The US government also has chimed in; on September 8, 2004, the US Food and Drug Administration (FDA) announced that "Supportive but not conclusive research shows that consumption of EPA and DHA omega-3 fatty acids may reduce the risk of coronary heart disease." This "Qualified Health Claim" from the FDA is significant as it was the result of petitions from manufacturers of omega-3 fatty acid products. FDA reviewed published scientific data and based its conclusions on the outcome of the review, which was extremely favorable towards the potential benefits of fish oil consumption for cardiovascular health.

Fish Oils and Brain Health

The brain is 60% fat by weight. Of this, between 25-30% is the omega-3 fat DHA, the most abundant fatty acid in neural tissue.[13] This highlights the importance of adequate DHA intake for brain health. The omega-3 polyunsaturated fatty acids of fish oil are incorporated directly into the membranes of brain cells. There, they facilitate cell-to-cell communication. Since communication is an essential aspect of nerve cell function (without which message transmission would be impossible), fish oils enhance your ability to use your noggin.

How do Brain Cells Talk?

Brain cells ("neurons") are not like chips in a computer – they must pool their information. No one brain cell holds all the pieces – and every decision requires input from thousands of individual cells, communicating chemically through their cell membranes. Those communication channels between brain cells must be composed of the right mix of fatty acids that allows them to correctly interpret the chemical messages ("neurotransmitters") they exchange.

Published research in humans shows that if you reduce the ease and efficiency of communication between neurons (disrupt cell-to-cell communication), you will reduce your ability to form and retrieve memories, learn and think logically.[14] Faulty membranes foster communication breakdowns – manifested, for example, as an inability to remember where those pesky keys are.

Fortunately, help is available. Studies show that facilitating the incorporation of healthy omega-3 fats into neuron cell membranes by increasing their dietary intake supports cell-to-cell communication abilities in the thinking and memory areas of the brain.

Supporting cell-to-cell communication may also increase memory capacity and decision making ability. A study published in the *American Journal of Clinical Nutrition* showed that in men and women more than 65 years old, as fish consumption and fish oil supplement intake increased, so did IQ, short-term memory ability and hand-eye coordination.[15] In other words, the more fish and fish oils in the diet, the longer these subjects retained better mental capacity.

The connection between fish oils and cognitive functions was confirmed in another study published more recently in the *Archives of Neurology*.[16] These medical researchers found that eating cold-water ocean fish just once a week dramatically promoted retention of memory capacity and decision making ability. Other researchers have also reported that the routine long-term daily consumption of at least 1000 mg of combined EPA and DHA successfully maintained thinking and decision making abilities in men and women 45 to 70 years old.[17] Furthermore, evidence collected from the landmark Framingham Heart Study suggests that just 180 mg of DHA taken daily (the equivalent of nearly 2.7 servings of fish per week) significantly enhanced and maintained cognitive function and mental acuity in this elderly population.[18]

And How Are We Feeling Today?

Diet and mood are intimately interconnected. After all, our guts are also known as our second brain. The guts and brain are formed from the same tissue during embryonic development. In addition, there is a network of nerves and neurotransmitters lining the guts and has direct linkages to the brain. Feelings and moods can have direct effects on digestive function, and foods we eat can have mood and mind-altering properties. Given the extent to which omega-3 fats are involved with cognitive function, it also makes sense that there would be an important link between fish oils, brain chemistry and mood.

> *"…routine long-term daily consumption of at least 1000 mg of combined EPA and DHA successfully maintained thinking and decision making abilities in men and women 45 to 70 years old."*

The abilities of omega-3 fatty acids from fish to promote a positive outlook have been confirmed in a study published in the *American Journal of Clinical Nutrition.*[20] It was found that men and women over 60 years old with lower long-term intakes of fish oils exhibited more negative emotions than were expressed by others who regularly consumed more fish oils (as fish or as supplements). This result echoes the interesting finding reported in the *British Journal of Psychiatry,* which showed that across the globe, the likelihood of good mental health and a positive attitude toward life increases with increasing fish (and fish oil) intake.[21]

Fish oil isn't just for adults. It also seems to enhance mood in children. According to research published in the *American Journal of Psychiatry,* the intake of fish oil in the form of approximately 400 mg of EPA and 200 mg of DHA taken daily in a trial lasting for 16 weeks showed significant improvements in mood at eight weeks, continuing on through the end of the study at 16 weeks.[22] It certainly seems that fish is good mood food.

Fish Oils and Healthy Vision

None of the parts of your visual system – lens, retina or optic nerve – can function without large amounts of omega-3's, especially DHA. In fact, even when we're in a fasting state, the eye retains its DHA at the expense of using other parts of its retina for energy and other chemical functions. Of the fatty acid content of the retina, researchers estimate that 50-60% is in the form of the extremely beneficial DHA. Omega-3 fatty acids may play a major role in maintaining healthy vision and ocular function.

The Oil that Sharpens Vision

It's been known for years that the highest visual acuity requires the presence of enough DHA to facilitate the chemical reactions of the visual cycle that ultimately result in a message sent through your optic nerve to your brain's visual image interpretation center. Both the retina and the optic nerve need large amounts of DHA in an uninterrupted supply.

In addition to translating light into visual images, the chemical reactions of the visual cycle generate very large amounts of oxidizing by-products, or free radicals.[23]

Adequate amounts of DHA, obtained through the circulation from the diet and dietary supplementation, will perform antioxidant functions within the eye and optic nerve and will defend the eye and related structures against uncontrolled free-radical oxidation. An interesting study published in *Investigative Ophthalmology and Visual Science* revealed that supplementing the supply of DHA available to the retina supports the antioxidant activity within retinal neurons and promotes healthy vision.[23] The antioxidant actions of DHA benefit the entire eye and protect the function of its vital components.

"Supplementing the supply of DHA available to the retina supports the antioxidant activity within retinal neurons and promotes healthy vision."

Further research shows that a high intake of omega-3 fatty acids from fish also supports the health of the macula. The macula of the eye is near the center of the retina and contains a high concentration of cone cells, which play a significant role in central vision. Researchers have conducted a meta-analysis of studies that was published in the journal *Archives of Opthalmology*. An evaluation of published studies led scientists to conclude that the consumption of 2 or more servings of fish per week and high intakes of their omega-3 oils seemed to play an important role in protecting macular function.[24] Of course, as the authors mentioned, additional randomized controlled trials are needed to fully assess the effects of omega-3 intake on macular health, However, the results of this analysis were extremely promising. Ensuring optimal omega-3 fatty acid intake, with a particular emphasis on DHA, can lead to promotion of healthy visual function as we age.

Fish Oils and the Immune System

A huge and ever-expanding body of reliable scientific evidence consistently indicates that the fish oils work to promote a stable immune system. All of the evidence points in the same direction: fish oils promote the optimal balance between the production of compounds that stimulate hyper-reactivity of the human immune system and the production of compounds that ensure optimal effective responses. In other words, this modulating activity of fish oils promotes a normal, healthy immune response. This conclusion was confirmed by the results of a study published recently in the *Journal of Clinical Endocrinology and Metabolism*. The study assessed the relationship between levels of polyunsaturated fatty acids, as found in fish oil, and circulating immune factors The researchers confirmed that the higher the concentration of fatty acids found in fish oil you consume, the more well-balanced your immune system will become.[25]

Fish Oils and Healthy Skin

Skin cells, like other cells throughout the body, have cell membranes composed of lipid bilayers that facilitate cellular communication, leading to an inflow of nutrients and an outflow of toxins. This exchange is necessary for promoting the health of these and all cells. On the skin, the manifestations of dysfunctional or unhealthy cells become obvious since the skin is an area that is exposed to the outside world. Keeping these cells happy, supple, and vibrant means reaping the benefits of healthy skin. Of course, this is everybody's goal. But whether your skin can function properly while remaining healthy looking and attractive is largely determined by what you eat. Like every other part of your body, your skin will reward you for treating it well. And, like every other part of the body that has been examined, your skin loves, needs, and wants the healthy omega-3 fats that are provided by fish oils.

Your skin is exposed to the harshness of our environment on a daily basis. This exposure poses major challenges. The consumption of fish oils helps maintain your skin's youthful vibrancy and suppleness while strengthening the protection it provides as the body's major external organ. Research summarized in an article published in the *American Journal of Clinical Nutrition* found that daily intakes of several grams of fish oil every day can promote healthy skin.[26] Because "healthy skin" promotion by the fish oils depends in part on the natural state of the skin, it is likely that the skin of fair-skinned individuals will benefit the most from supplementation of the diet with fish oils. Fish oil and the omega-3 fats contained within it enhance the functionality of the skin as an immune barrier by facilitating nutrient exchange and toxin removal within cells.

Of course, another mechanism of skin support by omega-3 fats is through modulating the production of chemicals by the immune system in response to certain exposures. As reported in research published in the *Journal of Lipid Research* decades ago, it is not healthy for the skin to be exposed to increased production of pro-inflammatory triggers.[27] However, within the skin, fish oils help to maintain a healthy balance of pro-inflammatory and anti-inflammatory metabolic compounds. You can nurture your skin by ensuring that cold-water ocean fish and fish oils are part of your daily diet.

Fish Oils and Healthy Joints

Flexibility and ease of motion are two characteristics of healthy joints. Due to the effects seen with fish oils on promoting a balance of the chemical messengers produced by the immune system, intake of fish oils has been shown to enhance normal joint flexibility and maintain ease of motion as we age. Fish oils also promote joint lubrication while maintaining joint comfort. In a study published recently in the journal *Nutrition,* the daily consumption of 3000 mg of fish oils was shown to enhance healthy joint movement and flexibility in a group of middle-aged men.[28] The results of this study confirm that healthy joints are simply more of the benefits to be obtained from installing fish oils as one of your cornerstones to Healthy Aging.

How Do I Know Whether I'm Consuming Enough of the Fish Oils?

The obvious way to know is that, usually, your body will tell you. You may notice a difference in your health and well-being, that you feel well or your skin looks better.

Beyond that, there is a way your doctor can determine whether you are consuming enough of the fish oils. An article published in *Cardiovascular Research* describes a lab test that can determine your "omega-3 index."[29] This index is calculated by dividing the EPA + DHA content of a sample of your red blood cells by the total fatty acid contents of those cells. There's no need to guess – you can test your level of omega-3 fitness. In terms of having this testing done, check with your nutritionally informed physician or naturopathic doctor to see if they offer this analysis.

What about those Warnings Concerning Eating Too Much Fish?

Many of the recent warnings are based on the fact that many types of fish can have a relatively high concentration of mercury. Organic mercury poisoning is a very real threat, given the generally polluted condition of our planet's oceans, lakes and rivers. Analysis performed by the Midwest Center for Environmental Science and Public Policy, published in the *Journal of Nutrition* concluded that the daily consumption of at least 1000 mg of fish oils cannot be achieved solely from either farmed or wild-caught fish without increasing your risk for developing cancer (due to the level of contaminants in commonly consumed fish species).[30] The good news is that the benefits of omega-3 fatty acids can be attained safely through the daily consumption of a high quality, purified fish oil supplement. The emphasis needs to be placed on high quality products that are certified to be free of mercury and other pollutants and carcinogens. Check with the manufacturer to see if they have documentation showing that the batch used in the product has been tested for mercury and other toxins.

> *"...the benefits of omega-3 fatty acids can be attained safely through the daily consumption of a high quality, purified fish oil supplement."*

I've Heard Fish Oil Disturbs Digestion

Belching and a fishy aftertaste are common when crudely prepared fish oil supplements are consumed. These "side effects" are not caused by EPA or DHA but by other oily substances left in the supplements by the crude processing procedures. More highly refined fish oil supplements contain very little of the offending materials and do not cause noxious and inconvenient (not to say antisocial!) side effects. Again, using high quality products offers protection against these commonly experienced symptoms. In addition, taking your fish oil supplements with food reduces the occurrence of these unpleasant digestive issues.

Omega-3 Fish Oil

- Fish oils comprehensively support healthy heart and cardiovascular function.*
- Fish oils enhance the structure and function of cellular membranes.*
- EPA and DHA promote healthy brain development.*
- EPA and DHA support healthy cognitive funtion and enable efficient cell-to-cell function.*
- Fish oils support healthy circulation.*
- EPA and DHA may enhance healthy vision by promoting normal retinal function.*
- EPA and DHA promote vibrant and youthful skin.*
- Omega-3 fatty acids enhance the function of signaling patways in the human body.*
- Omega-3 fatty acids enhance the cellular uptake of vital nutrients.*
- Omega-3 fatty acids from fish oil protect brain tissues from the effects of oxidative damage.*

2

Vitamin D—More than just a Vitamin

How Can It Do So Much?

The discovery of vitamin D early in the 20th century eventually led to several important discoveries that have changed how nutritionists look at vitamins. Most importantly, under *ideal circumstances* of sun exposure, the human body can make all the vitamin D it needs without help from the diet. But, the amount of vitamin D produced in the body depends on the length of time and the amount of skin exposed to ultraviolet B sunlight – too little sunlight, too little vitamin D. If sunlight exposure is inadequate, vitamin D becomes a dietary essential that must be consumed in order to satisfy the body's needs. More recently, evidence has come to light regarding the widespread deficiency of vitamin D. While the majority of individuals deficient in this vitamin live in northern latitudes, where sun exposure is limited except in the summer, a number of studies report vitamin D-deficient populations in states and countries where sunshine is intense year-round. An important factor seems to be that the darker an individual's skin, the longer the sun exposure necessary to produce vitamin D. Vitamin D deficiency is common in

African Americans for this reason. Research also suggests that vitamin D deficiency may be common in India, a country where there is plenty of sunshine. What these facts tend to point to is sun-avoidance, even in the tropics, is contributing to this global epidemic of vitamin D deficiency. Dietary factors can impact vitamin D nutrition, as can possibly several factors that limit the conversion of vitamin D in the body to its active form.

Whether vitamin D is consumed through a fortified dairy food, is part of a dietary supplement or is synthesized in the skin in response to exposure to sunlight, these forms of vitamin D are inactive. They must undergo a 2-step activation process: step 1 occurs in the liver (converting vitamin D to 25-hydroxyvitamin D_3 or $25OHD_3$), step 2 is performed by kidneys and multiple other organs in the body to convert $25OHD_3$ to the most active form of the vitamin, 1,25-dihydroxyvitamin D_3 ($1,25(OH)_2D_3$). Although the rate of the renal activation step is controlled by other hormones in response to fluctuations in plasma calcium concentration, at $25OHD_3 2$ levels achieved by most modern humans, both the hepatic step and the production of $1,25(OH)_2D_3$ in multiple other organs depends directly on the amount of vitamin D produced by the skin or added to the blood through the diet. Only when $25OHD_3$ levels exceed 50 ng/ml, a level only achieved when adults take 5,000 IU per day or sunbathe regularly, does the metabolism of Vitamin D become similar to other such hormones, controlled with feedback to limit production.

Although called a "vitamin," vitamin D actually is probably better characterized as a "prohormone" that becomes a full-blown hormone after the sequential activation steps. Vitamin D also differs from most other vitamins in another important respect. Typically, vitamins assist other molecules (usually enzymes) to do their jobs. In contrast, vitamin D does not participate in any other molecules' functions. Instead, vitamin D interacts with messenger molecules to signal to a cell's DNA that it needs to switch on or off a particular cell function.

Traditionally it has been believed that the functions controlled by vitamin D all involved the absorption of calcium and phosphorus by the intestinal tract and the regulation of the amounts of these minerals in the blood. These tasks require fully activated vitamin D $(1,25(OH)_2D_3)$ to help control the rates of dietary calcium absorption, bone formation and resorption in the skeleton and excretion of calcium by the kidney.

Beyond this, when $1,25(OH)_2D_3$ is made in tissues, it becomes an autonomous activator of more than 1,000 genes, thus vitamin D influences processes in organ systems throughout the body.[1] Since the functions of vitamin D in multiple tissues are autonomous, it has as many mechanisms of actions as genes it regulates. [2] These autonomous hormone actions, termed *autocrine* or inside the cell, extend far beyond the regulations of calcium and phosphorus levels, and these exciting functions of vitamin D are just now beginning to be untapped by researchers. As a nutrient, vitamin D has the potential to be a game-changer and, with more research, the vast reach of this health-giving essential nutrient will begin to be realized.

The Sun, the Skin and Vitamin D

Skin production of vitamin D is determined by length of exposure to sunlight, latitude, season, amount of skin exposed, height of the sun in the sky, the amount of air pollution, and degree of skin pigmentation. The reason vitamin D is considered to be a vitamin is that there is virtually no way most of the world's population living in non-equatorial areas of the globe can be exposed to sufficient sunlight year-round to be able to make enough vitamin D in their skin to satisfy their metabolic needs. As the sun must be high enough up in the sky so your shadow is shorter than you are in order to make Vitamin D, additional vitamin D from fortified foods or dietary supplements is needed by almost everyone from birth throughout life.

The amount of vitamin D that is formed in the skin is proportional to sunlight exposure – greatest at solar noon (when the sun is as high as it will be that day). During the summer, at most latitudes, that means between 11 AM and 3 PM (local time) during the months with the longest day length. Likewise, the amount of vitamin D that is partially activated by its conversion to $25OHD_3$ by the liver is determined by the amount of vitamin D made by the skin and absorbed from the diet. Consistent with this concept, darker-skinned ethnic groups produce less vitamin D and therefore less $25OHD_3$ than do lighter-skinned individuals in response to the same degree of sun exposure. Similarly, effective sunscreen also prevents vitamin D synthesis in the skin, as do clothes. Fortunately, all adults are able to absorb supplemental vitamin D unless a disorder in fat digestion or absorption is present or inhibitors of fat digestion are present.

How Much Vitamin D Do I Need?

While the amount of vitamin D needed by any individual on a daily basis varies, it is clear that current reference amounts are woefully inadequate. Two recent studies published in the *American Journal of Clinical Nutrition* serve to highlight this point rather dramatically. The first study looked at the relationship between serum levels of vitamin D3 and blood levels of 25(OH)D, the functional status indicator of vitamin D and its principal storage form in the body.[3] What the researchers found was that a $25OHD_3$ blood level of 40 ng/ml was needed in order for the liver enzymes that are responsible for the conversion of vitamin D to become saturated in 50 % of people. This means that, up to this blood level, the body's needs for vitamin D are not adequately met in 50% of people, as all of the vitamin D available is quickly being converted and utilized by the body and those people are no longer suffering from "substrate starvation." When one achieves levels of 50 ng/ml, more than 90% of people are no longer "substrate starved." According to these researchers, the point at which the liver enzymes are saturated can be defined as the low end of "normal" vitamin D status. However, at this low level, the body is not storing any vitamin D for future use and is unable to adequately satisfy the burden of need for vitamin D by all organs and systems.

A second study looked at the amount of vitamin D needed on a daily basis by adults to raise the concentration of 25(OH)D to the minimum level of 30 ng/mL (which is considered to be sub-optimal). Based on the findings of this six-month randomized double-blind, placebo-controlled study, the researchers concluded that adults needed to take between 3,800 and 5,000 IU daily for 97.5 % of people to obtain this minimum concentration.[4] An earlier study of 208 African American women by the same research team found that a daily dose of 2,000 IU of vitamin D3 failed to raise levels of 25(OH)D to above 30 ng/mL in 40% of the participants. These findings formed the basis for conducting the new study in African American and white men and women. While the higher dosages administered in the new study successfully brought the majority of study subjects up to the minimum threshold 25(OH)D level of 30 ng/mL, researchers found that many African American subjects required a daily dose that was 50% higher than the white study subjects in order to achieve this goal. This indicates that certain individuals and groups require much higher intakes of vitamin D to optimize health.

These studies also illustrate the fact that the current Recommended Daily Allowance (or "RDA") of 400 IU for all adults fails to even come close to meeting daily vitamin D requirements. Regardless of age, ethnicity and other factors, this amount just doesn't cut it given the evidence and recent data concerning widespread deficiencies. Children are also at risk for being low in vitamin D. Vitamin D deficiency in children is usually seen when blood levels are tested, and many are severely deficient.

It had earlier been thought that excessive supplemental doses of vitamin D may lead to signs of toxicity. There have been scattered

> "…the researchers concluded that adults needed to take between 3,800 and 5,000 IU daily for 97.5 % of people to obtain this minimum concentration."

reports of toxicity to vitamin D in the literature but these all are either dosing errors, rare industrial manufacturing errors, or from the administration of high doses of Vitamin D2 by physicians. However, most of these reports have been affiliated with vitamin D2 supplements taken at high doses. Vitamin D2 is produced synthetically and is the form that occurs in plants. Vitamin D2 is generally safe at normal doses; however, it is considerably less efficient at being converted to the active form of vitamin D in the body. Vitamin D2 is also not human vitamin D as it does not occur naturally in the body, and its metabolism may result in byproducts that are not normally found in humans.[2] The consensus now is that vitamin D3 (the form found in humans and other mammals) is the optimal form of vitamin D for supplementation and is extremely safe even at higher doses. Vitamin D3 is more effective than vitamin D2 at raising levels of 25(OH)D, the standard laboratory measure of vitamin D sufficiency.

Most scientists agree that the existing recommendation for daily vitamin D intake is flawed because it is based on survey data that were interpreted with the assumption that vitamin D deficiency is virtually nonexistent in the United States. As mentioned above, vitamin D deficiency is highly prevalent worldwide, including in the US. Therefore, this assumption is blatantly incorrect. In her summary of the Experimental Biology 2004 Symposium on Vitamin D Insufficiency that was published recently in the *Journal of Nutrition*, the US Food and Drug Administration's Mona S. Calvo described "the pressing need to define a new dietary requirement for vitamin D" in light of "the widespread prevalence of vitamin D insufficiency in North America."[5]

Vitamin D Deficiency – More Prevalent than we think

Five years ago, in his 2003 Robert H. Herman Memorial Award in Clinical Nutrition, Dr. Michael F. Holick argued convincingly that there is an unrecognized epidemic of vitamin D deficiency among children and adults in the US.[6] In children and adults, vitamin D deficiency results in bone issues – issues that are on the rise in 21st century America. In fact, Dr. Holick's research published in the *Journal of Clinical Endocrinology and Metabolism* discovered that at least half of all adult women in the US do not consume even 400 IU of vitamin D daily.[7]

Other scientists who have published their research results more recently in the *Journal of Nutrition* have made the same discovery: about 25% of all adult men and over half of all adult women in the US do not consume even 400 IU of vitamin D daily.[8,9,10] These percentages are doubled among black and Hispanic men and women. Even more adults are vitamin D "insufficient" – a fancy way of saying that they haven't reached the low levels associated with clinical deficiency but have lower than optimal levels, nonetheless.

Vitamin D Levels and Normal Aging

While the consumption of lower levels in youth may allow one to achieve better blood concentrations of vitamin D, the requirement increases in middle age and thus the dose required to achieve optimal levels also increases. For one thing, the ability of your skin to make vitamin D in response to sunlight becomes much less efficient – skin loses 50% to 75% of its ability to make Vitamin D in response to exposure to sunlight by age 60 – increasing the need for dietary vitamin D to narrow the ever-expanding gap between vitamin D requirement and supply. For another, older people tend to spend less time exposed to the sun – partly out of fear of skin cancer, partly out of reduced mobility. In addition, the ability of the kidneys and tissues to perform the final step in the activation of 25-hydroxyvitamin D_3 to 1,25-dihydroxyvitamin D_3 declines with age, meaning that even more vitamin D must be available in the blood in order to satisfy the physiological needs of the calcium economy for the older adult. Finally, overweight individuals need to consume more vitamin D than they needed when they were lean and trim because fat deposits soak up and store vitamin D – the more fat, the greater the percentage of ingested vitamin D that ends up in storage rather than use.

What If Vitamin D Recommendations were linked to the Vitamin's Functions – Instead of Surveys and Assumptions?

Many scientists now think that one way to ensure that someone's vitamin D health is optimized is to recommend that the person consume enough vitamin D to prevent more than a trickle of parathyroid hormone (PTH) from being released by the parathyroid glands. PTH is selected as the biomarker for vitamin D adequacy because the parathyroid glands secrete PTH when they sense that the concentration of calcium in the blood is getting too low to be able to support brain and heart muscle function. PTH is the hormone that 1) triggers renal conversion of $25(OH)D_3$ to $1,25(OH)_2D_3$ in order to increase the efficiency of absorption of dietary calcium (usually only 20% to 40% of ingested calcium is absorbed so there's plenty of room for improvement) and 2) itself causes bone tissue within existing bones to dissolve in order to add to the circulating supply of calcium. If vitamin D keeps the plasma calcium level high enough, the parathyroid glands sense that there is no need for them to secrete PTH – and less bone is destroyed in order to release its calcium. However, other biomarkers like PTH exist, and scientists are discovering that other biomarkers, such as the amount required so that breast milk has enough Vitamin D for the infant, require even high vitamin D blood levels to be satisfied, 7,000 IU/day in the case of breast feeding women.

Findings published recently in the *Journal of Nutrition* have shown conclusively that the density of skeletal bone begins to decline just when vitamin D intake becomes too low to prevent an increase in PTH secretion.[11] On the other hand, recent findings published in the *Journal of Bone and Mineral Metabolism* demonstrate that the first measurable indicator of early vitamin D deficiency in adult human's blood is an increase in PTH secretion.[12] As confirmed by the results of studies published recently in the *Journal of the American Medical Association* and the *Journal of Clinical Endocrinology and Metabolism*, minimizing parathyroid secretion of PTH by optimizing vitamin D intake achieves a true healthful balance between the diet, vitamin D, calcium and the skeleton.[13,14]

So How Much Vitamin D Do I Need?

A steadily growing body of scientific research demonstrates that daily intakes of vitamin D much greater than the current RDA of 400 IU are required to minimize PTH secretion, optimize skeletal health, and perform the myriad of other functions inside the cell. For example, the results of an elaborate analysis of published research in the *Journal of the American Medical Association* (*JAMA*), indicate a clear improvement in bone health among men and women over 60 years of age who routinely consumed double the RDA (about 800 IU of vitamin D daily) compared to those who stuck to the RDA.[15] In fact, the results of the Women's Health Initiative Study published recently in the *New England Journal of Medicine* proved that the RDA for vitamin D was no better than vitamin D deficient diets in protecting the skeleton.[16] The results of another study published recently in the *British Medical Journal* indicate that even 800 IU daily is not enough vitamin D for every elderly person to help prevent falling and fractures.[17]

"...daily intakes of vitamin D much greater than the current RDA of 400 IU are required to minimize PTH secretion, optimize skeletal health, and perform the myriad of other functions inside the cell."

The best estimates available suggest that an intake of 2,000 IU of vitamin D per day is the bare minimum that should be consumed by adults who also expose themselves to full-body sun on the weekends, just to ensure that the body's daily needs are met. A pioneer of vitamin D research, Dr. Hector F. DeLuca of the University of Wisconsin, has advised all adults to consume 2000 IU of vitamin D daily.[15] However, remember studies suggest that an intake of between 3,800 IU and 5,000 IU of vitamin D3 are needed on a daily basis to achieve levels of 25(OH)D3 of 30 ng/mL in 97.5% of people.[4] Many researchers, including Dr. John J. Cannell, Director of the Vitamin D Council, have suggested that optimal levels of 25(OH)D3 for health and wellness are 50 to 80 ng/ml[2] In order to obtain these levels, most adults require a daily intake of 5,000 IU of vitamin D3. Certain individuals (those with dark skin, obese, or older) may require even more. Taking 5,000 IU of vitamin D3 on a daily basis is very safe with little, if any, risk of toxicity. It has been suggested that everyone should be periodically tested for blood levels of twenty-five-hydroxy-Vitamin D [25(OH)D] to ensure that adequate concentrations are being sustained. The first test can be performed after 2 or 3 months on a daily dose of 5,000 IU, and then periodically thereafter. This is in fact the only way to ensure that you are getting the amount of vitamin D that your body needs to function optimally. Check with your nutritionally-oriented physician or naturopathic doctor in order to assure that your 25(OH)D levels are between 50 and 80 ng/ml, the mid point on the reference range.

Vitamin D – Not Just for Good-Looking Bones

Although you and your doctor may not know this, very reliable hard-core research (most funded by the US government) has demonstrated that without a doubt, failing to consume enough vitamin D will increase your chances of developing several chronic conditions.[6]

As important as it is to consume enough vitamin D to maximize intestinal calcium absorption and minimize PTH secretion, much more Vitamin D is necessary to supply enough 25-hydroxyvitamin D_3 to the brain, heart, small intestine, colon, prostate, breast, lung, stomach, pancreas, skin, testes, ovaries, parathyroid gland, macrophages, lymphocytes, bone marrow and other organs and tissues to allow them to perform their own local conversion of 25-hydroxyvitamin D_3 to 1,25-dihydroxyvitamin

D_3.[6] In fact, locally-produced 1,25-dihydroxyvitamin D_3 is now known to support many physiologic functions in these organs and tissues that are not related to bone health, including regulation of normal blood glucose metabolism, regulation of lymphocyte function, stabilization of heart muscle contractions, normalization of inflammatory responses, production of naturally occurring antibiotics called antimicrobial peptides, promotion of healthy thyroid function, and hundreds of other functions. For example, a 20-year study of 83,779 female nurses (the Nurses' Health Study) found that women who consumed the RDA for calcium plus at least 800 IU of vitamin D daily were very much more likely to have healthy blood sugar levels when these nutrients were consumed as a part of their diet.[19]

Vitamin D – Promoter of Mature Behavior in Young Cells

One of the most important functions of 1,25-dihydroxyvitamin D_3 throughout the body is its ability to force young cells to "grow up," called cellular differentiation. Because nature has decided that a cell can either reproduce itself or mature into its full function, all young cells face a choice: reproduce or go to work. Activated vitamin D (1,25-dihydroxyvitamin D_3) forces a cell to choose maturity and function instead of immaturity and continued replication. This tutelage by vitamin D ensures that there are enough working cells to keep any organ or tissue healthy.

Vitamin D keeps cells healthy and in a working state, allowing them to keep functioning at a high level and doing their designated job. The results of the Health Professionals Follow-Up Study that was published recently have shown that routine daily consumption of about 1500 IU of vitamin D enhances the ability to maintain digestive tract, and particularly colon, health.[20] These results also predict that routine daily consumption of only 400 IU of vitamin D doesn't have the same effect and likely will not support a healthy digestive tract, confirming the results of earlier research and results obtained again in the Women's Health Initiative Study published recently in the *New England Journal of Medicine*.[21,22]

Vitamin D – Defender of Self-Recognition

The importance of vitamin D's contribution to a healthy immune system cannot be overstated. According to research published recently in the *Journal of Immunology* 1,25-dihydroxyvitamin D_3 acts within the immune system to reduce the activity of the subpopulation of lymphocytes (a type of white blood cell) that are the most prone to accidentally mistake one of your cells for an outside invader.[23] In other words, vitamin D focuses cells on performing their designated tasks and prevents them from overdoing it - truly a nutrient that works as an immune modulator. It promotes enhanced immune activity when necessary but protects the immune system from becoming overactive.

> *"Thanks to vitamin D, your immune system is able to distinguish friend from foe…"*

At the same time, locally produced 1,25-dihydroxyvitamin D_3 also stimulates the activity of the subpopulation of lymphocytes responsible for correcting any "mistakes" that have already occurred. Thanks to vitamin D, your immune system is able to distinguish friend from foe and take the appropriate actions by fixing what's needed to get your immune system to function at its best.

Vitamin D – Immune System Support to the Next Level

Activation of the beneficial health-protective activities of white blood cells is a crucial event in the rapid response that is often required of the immune system. Research published in the *Journal of Immunology* has shown activated vitamin D to be a powerful stimulant to the white blood cells that mount the first line of chemical defense during the initial phases of a heightened immune response.[24] This finding has been confirmed more recently by data published in the *FASEB Journal* and in

Science.[25,26] Both studies illustrate the effectiveness of vitamin D in maintaining optimal immune responses by targeting the activities of immune components.

Run Faster, Jump Higher!

A little-appreciated consequence of too little vitamin D is muscle soreness that can often result in sore legs and increased discomfort while walking or even standing up. Research findings presented at a June 2006 conference on bone health indicate that vitamin D is a powerful promoter of muscle health and function in older adults and the elderly. In this study, daily dietary supplementation with 3,000 IU of vitamin D for 6 months increased lower limb muscle strength in previously vitamin D deficient elderly men and women by an average of 20% – enough to restore mobility and improve their quality of life substantially.[27] We do not know if this would be increased even further if they took 5,000 IU/day. In addition, none of the supplemented subjects exhibited any signs of vitamin D toxicity after the 6 months of vitamin D supplementation and all exhibited minimization of PTH secretion, a proposed measure of vitamin D adequacy.

Keeping with this line of thought, research over several decades points to the ability of vitamin D to influence athletic performance. A recent review highlights the results of numerous studies dating back to the 1950s showing that ultraviolet light exposure improves athletic performance.[1] This interesting review also suggests that athletic performance has seasonal variations, peaking at times of the year when vitamin D concentrations are naturally higher and decreasing when vitamin D levels are seasonally lower. Vitamin D administration has also been found to increase muscle strength and the percentage of Type II (fast-twitch) muscle fibers in humans. Studies in the elderly have found that vitamin D can improve balance and reaction time. Given that vitamin D is known to affect the expression of more than 1,000 genes, these findings come as no surprise.

Vitamin D's Helper Nutrients

In order to work effectively in the body, vitamin D needs certain cofactor nutrients. Vitamin D is metabolized by enzymes of the Cytochrome P-450 system. These enzymes require magnesium to facilitate their function. Subclinical magnesium deficiencies are common because many of us do not eat enough of the foods that contain magnesium (green vegetables, nuts, and whole grains). Research supports the fact that a majority of Americans are magnesium deficient. Besides playing a role as a cofactor for numerous enzymes, magnesium plays other significant roles in the body, including supporting bone health, nerve transmission and muscle function. Magnesium also promotes cardiovascular function.

Some very important calcium proteins, called Vitamin K dependent proteins, need adequate amounts of vitamin K to work properly. Vitamin K promotes calcium formation in bone but prevents deposition in other organs. The best source of vitamin K is green leafy vegetables, like spinach and kale. How often do you eat those vegetables? Furthermore, research shows that K2, the preferred supplemental form of vitamin K, plays a large role in cardiovascular health in addition to its role in supporting bone health.

In addition to ensuring sufficient magnesium and vitamin K levels, vitamin D requires zinc to perform its designated functions. The Vitamin D Receptor is like a glove, and the base of the fingers of the glove is a zinc molecule. Thus, in those who are zinc deficient, vitamin D cannot function properly. Zinc deficiencies are common, especially in those who eat little meat.

Boron may be another key mineral for enabling vitamin D's beneficial biological effects. While little is known about boron, other than it is common in green vegetables, fruit and nuts, a number of studies have found that it is important for facilitating the actions of Vitamin D on the cell wall. Studies show many Americans get little Boron, again because green vegetables, fruit, nuts, and whole grains are not consumed as often as they should be.

Thus, the key to health remains 5,000 IU of Vitamin D a day and a healthy diet, one rich in colorful vegetables and fruits, whole grains, adequate protein, and cold-water fatty fish, a diet that is varied, containing many different foods, and one that is low in foods that contain "empty calories." For added insurance, everyone should be on a multivitamin containing sufficient levels of magnesium, vitamin K, zinc and boron, among the other essential vitamins and minerals.

Vitamin D – the Vitamin of the 21ˢᵗ Century

Recent times have seen a reawakening of interest in the utility of vitamin D. Increasingly, scientists are recognizing the plethora of health-promoting activities of this unique "prohormone". Acting as a master switch that turns genes on and off, the key to your genome, this nutrient is much more than a vitamin; vitamin D "directs" the play of life by influencing multiple facets of the genetic code to act as it should. And the production and metabolism of the vitamin slows with aging. Ensuring sufficient levels of this critical nutrient can go a long way in supporting optimal wellness. With all of the health factors that are influenced by vitamin D, and with more being discovered every day, this nutrient potentially holds more than just the golden key to healthy aging.

"...vitamin D "directs" the play of life by influencing multiple facets of the genetic code to act as it should."

Vitamin D

- Vitamin D is an important regulator of calcium metabolism and supports bone health by maintaining calcium balance.*
- Vitamin D and calcium supplementation supports muscle strength and function.*
- Vitamin D is a cofactor for the expression of hundreds of genes.*
- Vitamin D is crucial for cellular differentiation and it maintains healthy cellular function.*
- Vitamin D is a nutrient that modulates immune function and promotes a healthy immune defense.*
- Vitamin D helps your immune system perform its key defensive functions.*
- Vitamin D promotes immune function by influencing expression of vitamin-D dependent genes that regulate host defense.*
- Vitamin D plays a key role in the function of macrophages, which are part of the immune system's cellular defense network.*
- Vitamin D is an essential nutrient that helps keep the cardiovascular system healthy.*
- Vitamin D may also contribute to the ability to support blood pressure levels that are already normal.*

3

Polyphenols – The Keys to the Kingdom

Plants have been used as a health supporting tool since ancient times. The use of therapeutic botanicals transcends cultures. Traditional herbalists throughout the world spent time observing the phenomena presented by nature through the interactions plants had with predators and the varied conditions of their environments and discovered that plants were surprisingly adept at adapting to difficult situations. More often than not, plants found ways to survive and even thrive in harsh conditions. Putting two and two together, these observers found that what benefits plants, fruits and vegetables in their struggle to survive would also be beneficial for humans. These observations by great healers through the centuries have led to the explosion we've seen today in the use of herbal therapies to promote optimal health. Plants are full of health-promoting compounds including vitamins and minerals. But they contain compounds that are even more exciting in their potential to promote wellness - the class of compounds collectively known as *polyphenols*. That's right! Polyphenols have been used to promote health since time immemorial. These compounds have been the backbone of the wisdom of traditional systems of medicine and it's only now that modern science is beginning to untap the beneficial effects that nature has endowed these substances with.

You may have heard of some of the more highly publicized polyphenols, such as **quercetin, hesperidin, resveratrol, epigallocatechin-3-gallate** ("EGCG"), **caffeine, genistein** and the **soy isoflavones,** as well as the **anthocyanins** in berries. Others that you will be hearing much more about in the near future include **fisetin, hydroxycinnamic acid** and **galangin** from flower pollen. These are just a handful of the thousands of polyphenols that have been isolated. While polyphenols serve important roles in plants as a means of defense from predators, research is finding that these compounds have significant pharmacological activities.

Vitamins, minerals and other phytonutrients are amazingly talented craftsmen, sculptors, artists, engineers, communications experts and skilled technicians. Polyphenols, on the other hand, orchestrate, conduct, administer and direct the immense processes of life. They are increasingly recognized as the major active components in fruits and vegetables. As the individual polyphenols have been studied in detail, and compared to each other, it has become clear that each acts slightly differently in benefiting human health.[1] The beneficial outcome of this integrated cooperation is a vastly greater robustness and versatility in our abilities to respond to health-challenging situations and environmental insults. Healthier responses lead to healthier aging.

Polyphenols in Healthy Aging

The scientific literature provides a feast of detailed evidence that very strongly documents the vital importance of polyphenols to vibrant health in all of its forms – tremendous and ever-increasing research highlights the effects of polyphenols in the areas of heart health, immune system health and strength, skeletal health and function, nervous system health and longevity, and blood glucose regulation. In all of these activities the polyphenols act as creative and sensitive managers, directing and redirecting cellular activities toward greater health. They are masters of cell signaling processes.

Most polyphenols interact directly with cell receptors or enzymes. These interactions trigger intracellular reaction pathways that work to multiply the potency of each polyphenol molecule. For example, as shown in research published recently in *BMC Neuroscience*, the polyphenolic **soy isoflavones** interact with estrogen receptors in brain cells to stimulate changes in DNA activation patterns.[2] These interactions ultimately lead to potential cognitive benefits. Further evidence of the interaction of polyphenols with cell-signaling pathways comes from literature outlining the ability of these compounds to modulate the normal inflammatory process in the body. Research suggests that polyphenols interact with genes, proteins and enzymes in the body, in a fashion similar to a conductor of an orchestra, to support and maintain a healthy inflammatory response, preventing imbalances in this crucial component of the immune system. Unique to polyphenols is their ability to influence several cell-based pathways and molecules, making them important modulators of immune and inflammatory processes.[3]

"…tremendous and ever-increasing research highlights the effects of polyphenols in the areas of heart health, immune system health and strength, skeletal health and function, nervous system health and longevity, and blood glucose regulation."

Dietary polyphenols can exert their effects on intracellular reaction pathways separately, sequentially or in combination, and the effects of one polyphenol can complement and reinforce those of another. In fact, many investigators have reported that mixtures of polyphenols have profound effects on cardiovascular health, heart health, healthy blood pressure regulation, liver health and overall immune system strength.[4,5] However, it is clear that the activities of these compounds are synergistic. More important than individual polyphenolic compounds is the combined effect of several. Clearly, the cooperative nature of the polyphenols overrides the properties of any individual superstar.

Anthocyanins

Berries, especially blueberries, are known to be a good source of the polyphenol subclass known as **anthocyanins**. New research shows that the health benefits of the anthocyanins extend throughout the body.

In one of the more recent studies, the blueberry anthocyanin, *pterostilbene*, showed an ability to support the health of colon cells by protecting against the early loss of cellular regulation.[6] Because colon health and function is so absolutely dependent on tight and well-managed cellular regulation, this finding demonstrates just how powerful the anthocyanins are as promoters, supporters and managers of colon health.

The abilities of the anthocyanins to beneficially manage, direct and redirect the functions of the body's physiologic systems are not limited to any one (or even few) of those systems. Cognitive functions, all-important to healthy aging, are sustained and boosted by anthocyanins.

In tests using laboratory animals, anthocyanin-rich blueberry extract has been effective in protecting against age-related deficits in neuron-to-neuron signaling in the brain, with accompanying improvements in learning abilities.[7] In one study, in which aging rats were fed a standard diet supplemented with blueberry extract for 8 to 10 weeks, performance on an objective test of learning and memory depended on how much of the anthocyanin compounds were found in the rats' brains.[8] In other words, those rats that ate the largest amount of anthocyanin-containing blueberry extract accumulated the most anthocyanins in their brains. These animals had the best learning capacity and were found to perform the most accurately on this standardized assessment.

Exciting new research has shown that anthocyanins also promote the healthy function of non-neuron cells in the brain.

These cells support neural activity by protecting neurons from the damage that can be caused by environmental toxins, oxidizing byproducts of the normal intense level of metabolic activity in neurons or aberrant electrical signals. In short, these cells help maintain the health of the neurons. However, if they become overstimulated they can harm the very cells they are responsible for protecting by promoting free radical generation. Research published in the *Journal of Neuroscience Research* shows that blueberry anthocyanins help the supporting cells modulate their activity level and the intensity of their responses to various stimuli.[9] What this means is that anthocyanins support brain defenses and stabilize the brain's internal environment. Further evidence for the neuroprotective benefits of blueberry anthocyanins comes from a study in which rats were either fed a diet rich in blueberries or were placed in a control group. The rats were then injected with a chemical into their brains that led to a significant impairment of learning performance. Although all rats had significant decreases in their learning abilities, the group of animals receiving the blueberry extract performed significantly better at standardized learning tasks. Imaging results on the brains of rats fed blueberries also revealed significant protection of neurons versus rats in the control group.[10] Because of their high anthocyanin content, blueberries are therefore protective against the damaging effects of free radicals on brain cells.

> *"...anthocyanins support brain defenses and stabilize the brain's internal environment."*

Together, these findings indicate that the anthocyanins in blueberries are able to enter the bloodstream, travel to the brain and act within the brain to foster an internal environment that supports learning ability and memory retention – both highly desirable results for promoting healthy aging.

Bioflavonoids

The interactions between the members of a large sub-class of polyphenolic phytonutrients, the **bioflavonoids**, and human cells, tissues and organs have been studied in great depth. Many investigators have discovered and confirmed that when consumed in sufficient amounts, the bioflavonoids are positively associated with the health and function of many body systems.

The way some bioflavonoids work might be surprising. In many cases, they act to maintain the activation of normal body control mechanisms so that these systems do not go out of tune. Laboratory experiments have demonstrated that many bioflavonoids, such as **quercetin** in apples, **fisetin** in strawberries, **epigallocatechin-3-gallate** in green tea, **galangin** from flower pollen, **hydroxycinnamic acid** in broccoli and **genistein** in soy, maintain the internal life cycle regulation of the body's cells. This helps the body comply with its needs for normal cell turnover, replacement and renewal as, over the years, the body experiences the physical and biochemical "wear and tear" of daily life. It is the best means the body has to "sweep out the old" and make room for the new.

As shown by the results of recent published studies, bioflavonoids foster normal life cycles in human cells.[11,12,13] While abnormally long lifetimes may seem to mean healthier aging, in fact, normal life cycles help cells, tissues and organs stay healthy and fully functional longer – and in so doing, promote healthy aging. A normal life cycle for cells includes the process of living healthy and dying when their functionality and utility have come to an end. It is the process of normal life, repair, death and renewal of cells that leads to healthy organs and systems of the body. Thus, maintaining these normal processes is what leads to optimal health and an interruption of these functions can have disastrous consequences on the body.

Further benefits from increased dietary intake of bioflavonoids include the promotion of healthy cognitive function. In a recently completed and published study of rat brain functions fisetin (found in strawberries) was seen to increase the ability to recall old memories (by facilitating the process known as "long-term potentiation" with the hippocampus, the functional center of memory recall in rats and humans).[14] This outcome probably resulted from the combination of properties of fisetin: antioxidant, cell function stabilizer and neural network enhancer.

Although not completely understood yet, the actions of another bioflavonoid, **resveratrol** (from grapes), within the brain contribute to the promotion of healthy brain longevity. As reported very recently in *Bioorganic and Medicinal Chemistry* resveratrol in the brain prevents the formation of molecular aggregates that interfere with information transmission between brain cells.[15] By maintaining open channels of communication, resveratrol sustains healthy cognitive functioning.

> *"By maintaining open channels of communication, resveratrol sustains healthy cognitive functioning."*

Resveratrol also plays active roles in heart health. As shown in a report published recently in the *Journal of Molecular and Cellular Cardiology* resveratrol supports capillary function within the heart muscle, increasing the oxygenation of the muscle and its contractile efficiency.[16] Recent studies highlight several distinct mechanisms whereby resveratrol can offer benefits to cardiovascular health. Studies show that resveratrol is an inefficient antioxidant *in vitro*, that is, in laboratory studies. However, when studied *in vivo*, i.e. in living systems, resveratrol shows an amazing ability to scavenge free radicals. Research suggests that the cardiovascular-protective effects stem from three major mechanisms of action: antioxidant, inflammatory-support and support of nitric oxide release. Nitric oxide release is necessary for enhancing circulation and supporting the health and integrity of blood vessels. These mechanisms lead to several distinct benefits that can be attributed to resveratrol supplementation. Some of these effects include protection of lipids from oxidative damage, supportive effects on normal heart rhythms, relaxation of blood vessels, which supports healthy circulation, and a reduction in free radical effects on cardiac tissue.[17] Given these broad effects on cardiovascular health, resveratrol appears to hold promise as a polyphenol that provides long-term and comprehensive benefits for heart function.

Resveratrol is just one of the many heart-healthy polyphenols. The **catechins** in green tea are a subclass of polyphenols that includes epigallocatechin-3-gallate (EGCG) and that contribute to cardiovascular health by protecting the integrity of the interior lining of blood vessels. The results of a study published recently in *Cardiovascular Research* have shown that catechins function as antioxidants by inhibiting the secretion of certain enzymes by over-stimulated vascular smooth muscle cells which can be detrimental to the linings of blood vessels.[18] EGCG and other catechins from tea also regulate the production of nitric oxide, stimulating blood vessel health and vasodilation, ultimately promoting circulatory function. By doing so, catechins enhance blood vessel function and structure.

Tea consumption has also been found to be protective of heart function over the long-term. Studies suggest that higher tea consumption leads to better protection of cardiac function with age. Tea contains numerous beneficial polyphenols, including the catechin EGCG. Furthermore, tea rich in EGCG has been shown to support circulation and promote antioxidant activity.[19]

Cranberries are similarly considered one of the more heart-healthy fruits because of their high polyphenol content. Surprisingly, cranberries have a higher amount of total polyphenols per serving than blueberries, apples, red grapes or strawberries.[20] Cranberries are particularly high in flavonoids, and also contain a small amount of resveratrol. Research conducted on cranberries shows that they support the body's antioxidant defenses and protect cholesterol molecules from free radical damage. Laboratory research using cranberry powder found that it stimulated the major cellular antioxidant systems including superoxide dismutase, catalase and peroxidase. Studies in humans have found that the polyphenolics in cranberries increase antioxidant nutrient levels in the blood, increasing the protection of the cardiovascular system.

Several polyphenols show cardiovascular and supportive effects by working as antioxidants, supporting the body's normal inflammatory response, protecting lipids and cholesterol molecules from oxidative damage, and by directly influencing the function of the heart muscle. The consumption of a wide variety of polyphenolic compounds, including the ones mentioned above, can yield far-reaching benefits for cardiovascular wellness.

Polyphenols as Antioxidants

Several polyphenols have direct antioxidant effects. Others are metabolized by bacteria in our intestines. These metabolites are absorbed into the bloodstream and they influence cell-signaling processes that lead to immune-supporting effects and free radical-scavenging effects. Polyphenols are the most abundant antioxidants in the diet. Typically, the total dietary intake of polyphenols is about 10 times higher than the intake of vitamin C and 100 times higher that the intakes of vitamin E and carotenoids. By themselves, the anthocyanins often contribute more than half of the total antioxidant activity of the diet.[21]

> "Polyphenols are the most abundant antioxidants in the diet."

The polyphenols not only directly detoxify potentially oxidizing substances within the body, they increase the body's inherent antioxidant defenses. For example, an important mechanism by which polyphenols enhance antioxidant defenses in the body is through stimulating the synthesis of glutathione, the major antioxidant enzyme within human cells.[22] As antioxidants, polyphenols display a dual nature – directly blocking oxidation themselves and recruiting more natural defense systems into the fray.

A considerable body of scientific literature underlines the important role of combating oxidative stress in the maintenance of optimal cell, tissue, organ and body-wide healthy function. Although the complex relationships between antioxidant status and healthy aging are still poorly understood and are being studied intensively, it is clear that the polyphenolic phytonutrients protect cell constituents against oxidative damage by virtue of their powerful antioxidant potency. They also help prevent oxidation from occurring. New research findings published in *Clinical Chemistry* show that low-density lipoproteins (LDL) that have had resveratrol added to them by the liver are resistant to oxidation.[23] Unoxidized LDL can be removed from the body safely without harm to the cardiovascular system.[24]

Our ability to increase our own antioxidant prowess was recently demonstrated by the results of a study published in the *Journal of Nutrition*.[25] In this study, the greater the number of different fruits and vegetables in the diet, the more effective the mix was in improving the body's antioxidant status. Women who ate on average 8 servings a day of a broad range of fruits and vegetables, providing an array of polyphenolic phytonutrients, increased their antioxidant status more than women who ate on average 9 servings a day of just a few fruits and vegetables. This finding reinforces the message that the more diverse and polyphenol-rich the diet, the healthier one is likely to be. It also speaks to the fact that one should consume a variety of brightly colored foods for health. After all, a variety of polyphenols are responsible for the range of beautiful, bright colors seen in fruits and vegetables.

Polyphenols can be the champions of your antioxidant defense system – and the more polyphenols you consume, the stronger your defenses.

Polyphenols – More Reasons to Love Fruits and Vegetables

Polyphenols are large molecules with very complex structures. While it's their chemical complexity that makes polyphenols so biologically active in the human body, this feature also makes their absorption in the intestinal tract very inefficient. Some polyphenols (such as genistein and the soy isoflavones) must be processed by intestinal bacteria before they can be absorbed at all – meaning that a healthy colon is a prerequisite to obtaining health benefits from dietary polyphenols. A healthy colon needs lots of soluble dietary fiber – and there's no better source of the best colon-friendly dietary fiber than the polyphenol-rich fruits and vegetables – whole or powdered. Then, after being absorbed, many polyphenols must be activated in the liver – another organ that must be in top shape before the health benefits of polyphenols can be maximized. As you may have guessed already, the best promoters and supporters of liver health and function are the polyphenol-rich fruits and vegetables.

The Bottom Line

The more fruits and vegetables you eat, the more polyphenols you enjoy. And, "enjoy" is the key concept here – polyphenols abound in fruits, vegetables, fruit juices, tea, coffee, red wine, chocolate and high-quality polyphenol-packed beverages and drinks made using cold-processed nutrient- and phytonutrient-rich fruit and vegetable powders.

Fruits (especially berries) and vegetables – natural health-promoting foods packed with polyphenols, especially the bioflavonoids and anthocyanins – eat plenty every day.

Quercetin

- Quercetin is a nutrient flavonoid that helps normalize oxidative stress in the body.*
- Quercetin, a dietary flavonoid, contributes to the body's free-radical fighting war chest of antioxidants.*
- Quercetin provides antioxidant effects that help the body maintain cellular health.*

Resveratrol

- Resveratrol has antioxidant properties, allowing it to act as a cellular rejuvenant by protecting cellular membrane lipids from oxidative damage.*
- Resveratrol may have potent cardioprotective properties. Several lines of research suggest that resveratrol confers protective benefits to heart tissue, supporting normal heart function and promoting healthy heart rhythms.*
- Resveratrol may play a role as a neuroprotectant. Brain tissue is highly susceptible to oxidative damage, which results in premature brain aging. Resveratrol protects the integrity of brain tissue, which may lead to support of brain health and cognitive function.*
- Resveratrol has the ability to confer protection to muscles and other tissues throughout the body. Resveratrol supports muscle and tissue health in the face of less than optimal circulatory function. Resveratrol also may have the ability to optimize healthy circulation.*
- Resveratrol modulates the normal cell cycle and is a regulator of cellular function, promoting normal cellular development in tissues throughout the body.*
- As a healthy aging nutrient, resveratrol protects mitochondrial function in cells. As we age, mitochondria, the energy factories in cells, are highly susceptible to oxidative damage, slowing the efficiency of cellular functions. Resveratrol promotes mitochondrial health and has been shown in animal studies to normalize metabolic functions, leading to its recognition as a longevity-promoting nutritional factor.*

Pomegranate

- Pomegranate contains high levels of antioxidants and natural compounds which reduce the cell damage created by free radicals during oxidation.*

4

Hyaluronic Acid – The Molecule of Youth

Relatively new as a dietary supplement ingredient, hyaluronic acid has now been available for more than ten years. However, it has been used much longer than that as an injectable for supporting joint structure. Of course, the nutrient is indigenous to our bodies and present in connective tissues, nerves, brain tissue, and the skin. Hyaluronic acid is a complex molecule made up of two special sugars, N-acetyl-glucosamine and glucuronic acid. Hyaluronic acid disaccharides are produced and secreted in nearby tissue by cells in joint cartilage, synovial membranes, the cornea of the eye, tear ducts and skin. Wherever hyaluronic acid occurs it plays vital roles in maintaining the hydration and lubrication of that tissue.

Joints, Cartilage, Mobility and Nutrition

The cartilage tissue that covers the contact surfaces of joints is made up of mats of interwoven strings of special sugars and proteins. The electrical charges on these mats makes them very attractive to water molecules (water is highly charged – that's why it conducts electricity so well). Cartilage is spongy because its sugars attract water, which makes the mats swell. When the swollen tissue is squeezed, it absorbs the shock by releasing water into the joint space. Remove the pressure and the water streams back in, restoring the size and shape of the fully hydrated tissue.

Because they are subject to so much wear and tear, the mats are replaced regularly – each one lasts a little under a month in a young adult. In order to maintain balance, an old mat must be removed before a new one can replace it. Once our joints stop growing, they have to adjust their replenishment/replacement cycle in order to stabilize the amount of cartilage covering their contact surfaces. As we age, our cartilage becomes less and less able to adjust and this replenishment cycle goes out of balance. The result is that the mats begin dissolving earlier and earlier. In addition, new replacements are not made quickly enough. As the insertion of new mats falls behind the rate of removal of old mats, joint surfaces can normally become thinner as a result of the aging process and more susceptible to mechanical breakdown from normal everyday activity. Replenishing the joints with the nutrition they need to stay healthy becomes absolutely critical.

The Wear and Tear on Our Joints

You don't need to be unhealthy or be diagnosed with a medical condition to experience joint discomfort – just continue doing what you always do and eventually one of your joints will get cranky from the effects of normal wear and tear. Or perhaps you over-exert yourself during a sports activity or day-hike and feel it in your knees later that night. That didn't use to happen. However, now you're getting older. Things change with age. Whatever the case, this usually signals the need for extra care and supportive measures to maintain healthy joints – joints whose nutrients are not replenished or replaced on a regular basis eventually may not be able to catch up and function as well as they used to. Welcome to the process of normal aging.

There are two ways to help your joints last as long as possible – exercise and nutrition. Becoming more active helps maintain healthier joints as activity stimulates the renewal of connective tissue, bone and cartilage. Two recently published human studies have confirmed the roles of physical activity in joint health. One of these studies showed that if you don't use your joints, their cartilage covering tends to thin out on its own.[1] A second study showed that moderate exercise increases the thickness of joint cartilage and improves joint performance.[2] Active individuals have active (well-functioning) joints.

Just as important is to remember to nourish your joints. Joints are known to benefit from regular "feedings" (through eating well and through dietary supplementation) with fish oils, glucosamine, chondroitin sulfate and hyaluronic acid. You can think of hyaluronic acid as the cement that holds things together. Hyaluronic acid thus supports the normal structure of joint tissue. Feed your joints hyaluronic acid and they will reward you.

Hyaluronic Acid and Joint Mobility

Batches of hyaluronic acid are synthesized and assembled into long chains before being secreted by articular chondrocytes (cartilage cells) and synoviocytes (cells that live in the synovial lining of the joint capsule). Regardless of its source, hyaluronic acid can be incorporated into the load-bearing sugar/protein mats of joint cartilage.

As shown in research recently published in the *Journal of Physiology* the unique properties of the special sugars that make up hyaluronic acid attract water and are responsible for the cushioning properties of healthy joint cartilage.[3] Because the synthesis of its component sugars slows with age, the replenishment of hyaluronic acid within a joint also slows with age, creating an inevitable imbalance in the cartilage's replenishment/replacement cycle. As the contact surfaces of the joint cartilage become depleted of hyaluronic acid, they become chronically dehydrated and lose their vital cushioning hydrostatic properties.

> *"Feed your joints hyaluronic acid and they will reward you."*

A large volume of published scientific research has demonstrated that adequate availability of hyaluronic acid can promote joint health and function. These conclusions have been echoed most recently in a mathematical analysis of the body of published research, itself published in the *Journal of Family Practice.*[4] The strength of the evidence certainly argues in favor of adding hyaluronic acid to your personal Joint Health program.

Vision and Hyaluronic Acid

Hyaluronic acid is synthesized within the human eye and is secreted into both tears and the aqueous humor of the eye in its non-acidic form, hyaluronidate. On the ocular surface, tears with normal hyaluronidate content exhibit greater lubrication during blinks. Yet while the eyelid is still, hyaluronidate maximizes the thickness of the protective fluid covering the surface of the eye – another reflection of the special properties of hyaluronidate. Within the eye itself, hyaluronidate forms part of a web of large molecules that confer structural stability to the retina and help keep it attached to the underlying cell layers.

Both advancing age and dry eyes reduce tear production and the amount of hyaluronidate that is secreted in tears; complaints about burning, itching, a sensation of the presence of a foreign body, redness and heaviness of the eyelids are common. Hyaluronic acid replacement, via drop form, can promote normal eye functions, as shown by the results of a study published in the *British Journal of Ophthalmology,* which *assessed the effects of eye drops containing hyaluronic acid.*[5]

Research consistently demonstrates that the insertion into the eyes of drops containing sodium hyaluronidate several times daily decreases burning, dryness, "foreign body" sensation, itching and mucous discharge. At the same time, tear formation is increased. These tears help protect the cornea from environmental insults, indicating that hyaluronic acid acts both on the surface of the eye and within the eye.

The chemical process of vision produces a number of oxidizing by-products.[6] The gradual steady accumulation of oxidative damage interferes with the functions of all parts of the eye. The hyaluronic acid in tears acts as a powerful antioxidant that preserves the structure and function of the visual apparatus.[7]

Keeping Skin Healthy Longer with Hyaluronic Acid

Aging skin is characterized by a significant loss of elasticity coinciding with a reduced content of hyaluronic acid.[8] Because hyaluronic acid is the most abundant water-binding glycosaminoglycan in healthy skin, loss of hyaluronic acid results in decreased water content and loss of elasticity. In addition, loss of hyaluronic acid is accompanied by increased compaction of collagen fibers. Skin depleted of hyaluronic acid takes on a dry and wrinkled appearance, much like joints depleted in hyaluronic acid lose their ability to retain moisture, and thus have decreased cushioning and shock-absorbing ability.

"Hyaluronic acid contributes to the organization and structure of the skin by increasing the amount of water that is bound into the structure of the skin – the better hydrated the skin, the more flexible it is."

In contrast, enrichment of the dermal layer of the skin with hyaluronic acid optimizes collagen organization ("packing"). Hyaluronic acid also has been shown to promote intercellular communication, allowing cells to cooperate more efficiently in organizing the collagen they produce. Hyaluronic acid contributes to the organization and structure of the skin by increasing the amount of water that is bound into the structure of the skin – the better hydrated the skin, the more flexible it is.[9] In addition, hyaluronic acid enrichment supports the ability of new skin cells to replace old, further facilitating the restoration and maintenance of healthy skin.

When the skin is exposed to oxidizing chemicals or conditions (such as sunlight), the lipid structures of cell membranes are susceptible to increased rates of oxidative peroxidation.[10] Skin cells with membranes that have been oxidized shrink and deform, losing cell-to-cell contact and "leaking" increased amounts of evaporative water from the abnormal spaces between cells, causing dehydration of the skin and reducing its flexibility.[10]

As reported in a paper published recently in the *Journal of Pharmacology and Pharmaceutical Science* hyaluronic acid is a powerful antioxidant within the skin that acts to maintain skin health by preventing lipid peroxidation and by maintaining the normal level of hydration within the skin.[10] These properties of hyaluronic acid promote flexible and supple skin, making hyaluronic acid a vital component of your Healthy Skin Preservation program.

How Does Oral Hyaluronic Acid Work?

Traditionally, hyaluronic acid has been used as an injectable to promote joint health and support joint structure. There have also been questions regarding the absorbability of hyaluronic acid when taken orally. Research shows that oral hyaluronic acid is in fact absorbed and that it functions in at least three important ways. Hyaluronic acid is a large molecule with repeating subunits that, when taken orally, naturally goes through the process of digestion in the digestive tract. Studies show that 1) A portion of the hyaluronic acid is absorbed intact, 2) A portion of it is broken down into its component sugars and absorbed in this way (providing building blocks the body can use to remanufacture hyaluronic acid, and 3) Hyaluronic Acid acts to stimulate the growth of beneficial bacteria in the digestive tract, which promote immune system health and lead to overall health of the joints, skin and connective tissue throughout the body. These three unique and distinctly separate mechanisms of activity illustrate the ability of oral hyaluronic acid to benefit and support the body's connective tissue.

To reaffirm the efficacy of oral hyaluronic acid for joint support, let's look at the results of an important Japanese study. This study, which was published in 2008, was carried out to assess the efficacy of oral hyaluronic acid in promoting healthy joint function and mobility. Fifteen individuals with achy knees were supplemented with 240 mg of highly purified hyaluronic acid daily for twelve weeks. Positive results were evident after 4 weeks of supplementation as the individuals had significant improvements in knee joint function and comfort. The benefits continued throughout the duration of the study, showing that oral hyaluronic acid supplements are effective for promoting healthy joint function.[11]

Now that we know that studies affirm the effectiveness of oral hyaluronic acid, let's look at evidence supporting the three mechanisms of activity. Bioavailability studies in animals show that hyaluronic acid taken orally reaches joint tissue. Radioactively-labeled particles of hyaluronic acid were found to reach the skin, bone and joints of rats after oral administration, showing that a percentage of orally administered hyaluronic acid is absorbed intact.[12] A further percentage of hyaluronic acid taken as supplements is digested and broken down into its component molecules. These components are absorbed into the bloodstream, providing the body with the building blocks necessary to produce hyaluronic acid on its own, allowing it to replenish its own stores. Finally, a very interesting study was carried out in which rats were administered hyaluronic acid orally. Researchers found that the orally administered nutrient was fermented by gut bacteria as a source of nutrition. Hyaluronic acid was shown to act as a prebiotic, as it increased the level of *Lactobacillus* and *Bifidobacterium* species in the intestinal tract.[13] Taking these important studies into account, we can see that oral hyaluronic acid supplements have both direct and indirect effects in supporting the health of our joints, skin and connective tissue. Given its broad range of potential benefits, hyaluronic acid is a crucial and important nutrient for healthy aging.

Top Reasons to Add Hyaluronic Acid to Your Healthy Aging Program

Hyaluronic Acid supplementation can support the following beneficial effects on the body:

- Joint Flexibility and Mobility*
- Joint Health and Function*
- Healthy Vision*
- Healthy Eyelid Lubrication*
- Skin Moisture and Elasticity from Within*
- Skin Vibrance and Fine Line Reduction*
- Attractive, Healthy Skin*

Hyaluronic Acid

- Hyaluronic Acid supports healthy joint flexibility and mobility.*
- H.A. promotes healthy synovial fluid and joint lubrication.*
- H.A. supports a healthy inflammatory response.*
- H.A. supports increased weight-bearing capacity of articular cartilage and joints.*
- Hyaluronic Acid supports protection from oxidative stress on joint tissues.*
- H.A. promotes the increased shock-absorbing capacity of joints.*
- H.A. supports the maintenance of healthy, strong connective tissue.*
- Hyaluronic Acid enhances the production of elastin in connective tissue, an important protein involved in connective tissue remodeling.*
- H.A. supports beautiful, supple, youthful-looking skin and vibrant, healthy hair.*

5

Pycnogenol® – Clinically Tested Breakthrough from France

(and air traveler's best friend)

The phytonutrients in **pine bark** have a long tradition of use in "folk medicine." The French explorer Jacques Cartier was introduced to tea made from boiling pine bark when Native Americans saved most of his crew from death by scurvy during the winter of 1534. In particular, the bark of the **French maritime pine tree** contains a distinct group of potent health-enhancing phytonutrients. These beneficial compounds, which include procyanidins, bioflavonoids and organic acids, are extracted from the bark by an automated, patented, multi-step procedure that avoids the use of potentially toxic solvents. The resulting water extract, patented and available as **Pycnogenol®**, is pure and contains no additives. Because the bark is grown layer by layer over a period of more than 30 years before it is harvested, there are neither seasonal nor annual variations in the composition of its ingredients, in contrast to other herbal extracts. Its purity, potency and consistency is thus unmatched by other phytonutrient-rich extracts. Pycnogenol® also has a tremendous amount of published research highlighting its many potential benefits.

The Link between Tree Bark and Human Health

The phytonutrients in Pycnogenol® are absorbed into the human bloodstream very rapidly and once there act as a team of very efficient antioxidants. While certain compounds may be absorbed unmodified, several of these nutrients are acted upon by the beneficial bacterial population of the gut and are absorbed into circulation. The antioxidant prowess of Pycnogenol® is evident from the fact that the consumption of as little as 50 mg of Pycnogenol® three times daily substantially increases the total antioxidant capacity (oxygen radical absorbance capacity; ORAC) of the blood of healthy adults. The measurement of ORAC capacity in human serum is a good indicator of the ability of nutrients to perform antioxidant functions in living systems - meaning the antioxidants are likely to have an effect where they are intended. New research published in *BMC Clinical Pharmacology* shows that five days of dietary supplementation with 200 mg of Pycnogenol® daily will stabilize elevated concentrations of antioxidants in the blood and that this increase in circulating antioxidant capacity can be maintained by continued supplementation with 200 mg daily.[1] In addition, research findings published recently in *Biomedicine and Pharmacotherapy* demonstrate that consuming 300 mg of Pycnogenol® even once produces powerful inhibition of cyclooxygenase enzymes in humans[2], supporting our normal inflammatory response and providing yet another explanation for the benefits of Pycnogenol®.

Pycnogenol® also recycles **vitamin C** and **vitamin E** after those vitamins have become loaded with stray electrons, preserving their essential antioxidant functions. Vitamin C is a major antioxidant inside and between cells and in the blood, and vitamin E is the single most important lipid-based antioxidant that is present in every membrane in every cell. The ability of Pycnogenol® to recharge these antioxidant vitamins gives you a huge advantage in your battle to control and minimize the effects of free radicals. Research also shows that, in addition to replenishing vitamins C and E, Pycnogenol® stimulates the production of antioxidant enzymes in cells themselves, which serves as an important first line of defense for them against free radical attack.

Pycnogenol Maintains Strong Antioxidant Protection and Vision

Enormous numbers of free radicals are produced within the eye (especially the retina) during the chemical conversion of light to sight. If free radical production remains unopposed, the normal processes of vision can lead to free radical overload, causing damage to the retina and cornea, which are particularly sensitive to oxidative damage. For this reason, structural components of the eyes are naturally rich in antioxidant nutrients. Often, these antioxidant stores may decline with normal aging, leading to changes in eye health. Pycnogenol®'s antioxidant abilities serve as an important buttress by shielding the eyes from the effects of excessive oxidative stress.

> *"...research shows that dietary supplementation with 50 mg of Pycnogenol® three times daily enhances retinal function and promotes visual acuity in the eyes of adult men and women, thus supporting healthy ocular function."*

In research published recently in the *Journal of Ocular Pharmacology and Therapeutics*, supplemental Pycnogenol® increased the activities of several antioxidant enzymes within the retinas of rats whose eyes were in a highly oxidizing environment.[3] Since Pycnogenol® was effective in animals. It is likely that Pycnogenol® will also have protective properties in healthy humans. Previous research had shown that Pycnogenol® protected fat molecules within the retina from oxidation by the free radicals produced during the visual cycle. By supporting retinal health, Pycnogenol® was shown to be a very powerful promoter of healthy eyes. In fact, research shows that dietary supplementation with 50 mg of Pycnogenol® three times daily enhances retinal function and promotes visual acuity in the eyes of adult men and women, thus supporting healthy ocular function.

Happy Blood Vessels and Well-Supported Peripheral Circulation

The circulation in the lower limbs can be effected over time as a result of free radical damage to the walls and valves of healthy arteries and veins. This may result in inefficient flow through these vessels back to the heart and throughout the body. The supply of oxygen and nutrients to the tissues may be disrupted and affecting the body's natural healing abilities.

Pycnogenol®'s antioxidants absorb and quench free radical electrons with great efficiency and can vastly maintain the resistance of small blood vessels and capillaries throughout the body to oxidative damage. The results of human clinical trials published recently in *Angiology*[4] and *Clinical Applications in Thrombosis and Hemostasis*[5] showed clear improvements in the ability of veins to expand and dilate, and blood flow and nutrient delivery to the lower legs with the consumption of 50 mg of Pycnogenol® three times daily for 4 to 6 weeks.

Further research shows that dietary supplementation with 150 mg of Pycnogenol® daily promotes optimal microcirculation in capillary networks of the lower legs in men and women.[6] A recently published study also found that taking 200 mg of Pycnogenol® daily was effective for reducing muscle cramps in healthy adults who experienced occasional cramps while consuming placebo.[7] These

> *"…consuming Pycnogenol® daily facilitates healthy blood flow and nutrient supply throughout the body.*

researchers yet again confirmed previous findings that consuming Pycnogenol® daily facilitates healthy blood flow and nutrient supply throughout the body.

Stay Healthy in the Air

Prolonged air travel has been associated with cardiovascular issues caused by inactivity (sitting in one place for extended periods of time) and dehydration.[8] Compression of veins by the edge of a seat could contribute to slowing of venous return of blood to the heart and pooling of fluid in the lower legs. Dehydration in an aircraft cabin also can cause some swelling in the lower legs. The inability to move freely combined with the subnormal air pressure and oxygen content within an airplane can also interfere with healthy circulation. Long airplane flights are especially concerning because of their prolonged nature and potential to have a greater impact on cardiovascular health.

Effective preventive measures while traveling include standing and stretching exercises, drinking copious amounts of water, and avoidance of tightly-fitting clothes, salty foods and alcoholic beverages.

Dietary supplementation with Pycnogenol®, which is rich in veno-supportive nutrients, can be highly beneficial. The results of a placebo-controlled clinical trial published recently in *Clinical Applications in Thrombosis and Hemostasis* suggest that every traveler should add Pycnogenol® to their travel preparations. In this study, 200 mg of Pycnogenol® or of placebo were consumed 2 to 3 hours before take-off and again after 6 hours in the air.[8] As opposed to the placebo, Pycnogenol® was found to be highly supportive of venous circulation during the flights – an indication that Pycnogenol® promoted circulation while supporting healthy vascular function within the adverse environment of an aircraft at high altitude for many hours.

Pay Attention, Please!

Several studies in recent years have looked at Pycnogenol®'s ability to support cognitive function, mood, and attention and concentration. A double-blind, placebo controlled pilot study was conducted in which 61 children aged six to fourteen years were given a daily dosage of 1 mg of Pycnogenol® per kilogram body weight or a placebo for four weeks.[9] The researchers found that Pycnogenol® intake for one month significantly enhanced concentration and attentiveness in these children. Scientists have suggested that these effects may be due to the antioxidant activity of Pycnogenol® and may also be a result of Pycnogenol®'s ability to enhance the production of nitric oxide, a molecule that supports increased circulation through arteries and veins, thus making it easier for nutrients to reach organs and systems, including brain tissue. In fact, further research on Pycnogenol® in children found that the same dose (1 mg per kilogram body weight) given over a one-month period increased total antioxidant status and was able to induce a highly significant increase in the level of reduced to oxidized glutathione in the blood.[10] As is widely known, glutathione is one of the most abundant antioxidants in cells throughout the body. What is interesting is that research shows that the lower the intracellular glutathione concentrations go, the faster cells (and hence tissues!) age. Glutathione is the key antioxidant protector of proteins, fats and DNA in cells. Maintaining glutathione concentrations in cells is critical for healthy aging. Even more important is ensuring that there is a healthy balance of the reduced glutathione to oxidized glutathione. The reduced form is crucial for glutathione's free-radical scavenging capability. Pycnogenol® recycles glutathione and keeps more of it in the free-radical attacking reduced form.

Pycnogenol® also has shown the ability to support memory function in the elderly. A study published in the *Journal of Psychopharmacology* highlighted research looking into the effects of Pycnogenol® supplementation over a three-month period on cognitive function and memory.[11] In this placebo-controlled trial, healthy elderly individuals were asked to take Pycnogenol® at a daily dose of 150 mg per day or placebo. The results of the trial showed significant benefits in memory function in the Pycnogenol® group after 3 months, indicating Pycnogenol®'s beneficial effect on cognitive function. Once again, researchers attribute this benefit of Pycnogenol® to its powerful antioxidant functions and its ability to protect brain cells from free radical damage.

Tree Bark and Human Health – Strong Links

Pycnogenol® - the unique water extract from the French maritime pine tree - has numerous tonic effects for the human body. This well-researched product deserves to be included as a core component of everyone's health and wellness armamentarium. Pycnogenol® reinforces the establishment of a healthy balance between oxidative stress and antioxidant capacity throughout the body. By doing so, Pycnogenol® is a strong and potent ally of visual health, vascular health, immune wellness and in the management of the inflammatory response, cognitive function and memory, and as a key nutrient for Healthy Aging.

Pycnogenol

- Pycnogenol® enhances protectin against the oxidative stress that accompanies aging.*
- Pycnogenol® supports healthy blood pressure levels anready within the normal range.*
- Pycnogenol® supports healthy cholesterol levels already within the normal range.*
- Pycnogenol® promotes healthy circulation.*
- Pycnogenol® supports immune and respiratory health.*
- Pycnogenol® supports joint and skin health.*
- Pycnogenol® enhances cardiovascular function and circulation.*

6

Green Tea – Drinking Your Way to Health and Longevity

Tea made from the leaves of the *Camellia sinensis* plant has been consumed for over 5000 years. After water, tea is the most popularly consumed beverage worldwide. Europeans, North Americans and North Africans drink mainly black tea, Asians seem to prefer green tea, and oolong tea is popular in China and Taiwan.

Tea is tasty, soothing and either warming or cooling (depending on whether you drink it hot or cold). But tea is so much more than that – it is a well-recognized enhancer of the health and performance of your heart, your cardiovascular system, your muscles, your teeth and your bones – just to name a few reasons why this natural food is so beneficial.

What Difference Does the Color of Tea Make?

Whatever its color or name, all true "teas" are produced from the leaves of the tropical evergreen plant, *Camellia sinensis*. When tea leaves are converted into black tea, the harvested leaves are allowed to ferment before and while drying – an oxidation process that changes both the color of the leaves and the nature of their phytochemical contents. In contrast, the leaves for green tea are steamed to prevent oxidation and phytonutrient change during drying. Oolong tea is produced by allowing a partial oxidation of the leaves, making oolong tea equivalent to "half-green and half-black" tea. About 20% of the tea produced worldwide is green tea. Essentially, then, with changes in the phytonutrient profiles, drinkers of the different types of tea can experience differing beneficial effects. Each phytochemical has unique healthful properties and, as antioxidants, has affinities for different types of free radicals.

What Does Green Tea have that is missing from Other Beverages?

Tea is a rich source of "**polyphenolic phytonutrients**." While this class of phytonutrients is huge, with over 4000 known members, tea leaves become heavily loaded with one particular class of phytonutrient during their growth. In unoxidized, unfermented green tea leaves, this class, the catechins, includes epicatechin (EC), epicatechin-3-gallate (ECG), epigallocatechin (EGC) and epigallocatechin-3-gallate (EGCG). During the oxidation process of converting green tea to black tea, the catechins also are oxidized, changing into a class called the **theaflavins**: EC becomes **theaflavin**, ECG becomes **theaflavin-3-gallate**, EGC becomes **theaflavin-3í-gallate** and EGCG becomes **theaflavin-3,3í-digallate**.

It has been estimated that one cup of brewed green tea contains between 100 and 150 mg of catechins, of which about half is EGCG and a little less than half is EGC. The other catechins are present but in much smaller amounts. Hot water extraction (brewing) maintains these relative proportions; EGCG comprises about half of the dissolved solids in brewed green tea.

Does the Source of the Tea Matter?

The exact amounts of the catechins and theaflavins that are present in any sample of tea,(green, black or oolong) depends on where the leaves are grown and just how the leaves are processed prior to drying. Of course, factors such as the soil the tea is grown in can influence the content of polyphenols. In addition, whether the tea is decaffeinated, blended or freeze-dried ("instant") and the specifics of its preparation (how much tea is used per cup or glass, how long the tea is left to steep, brew or dissolve, and at what temperature) all affect the resulting beverage's phytonutrient content. The process of decaffeination removes some of the phytonutrients along with the caffeine (an unavoidable consequence of the chemistry of decaffeination).

Brewed hot tea contains the largest amount of phytonutrients, "instant" teas have lost about 80% of their phytonutrients and "iced" and other ready-to-drink tea products contain even less. Diluting tea with milk, water or ice obviously reduces the amount of phytonutrients contained in each cup or glass. Interestingly, recent studies have found that taking tea with milk may reduce its ability to enhance blood circulation and hinder some of its antioxidant benefits. It's also important to realize that so-called "herbal teas" really are not "teas" but are boiled decoctions of the herbs used to make them – and they contain none of the beneficial tea catechins or theaflavins, although they certainly do contain beneficial compounds present in the particular herbs.

Tea as a Dietary Supplement

Why is all this important to you? It is important for you to remember that even though drinking tea is an extremely healthy practice, hot or cold teas prepared from either loose dried leaves, powdered leaves or "bags" are less reliable sources of tea phytonutrients than are the standardized powders used in the highest-quality dietary supplements. Standardized extracts control for the level of collective and individual tea polyphenols, and research shows that in order to receive optimal benefits from tea intake, an optimal amount of polyphenols needs to be consumed on a daily basis. This could mean drinking cups and cups of tea per day. In addition, the catechins in high-quality standardized powders are absorbed about twice as readily as they are from teas.[1]

Of course, when it comes to drinking tea, sometimes enough can be enough! And some days you'd just rather drink something else. Not to worry – combining tea (or even replacing tea as a beverage) with a top-of-the-line dietary supplement high in catechin content is the perfect answer. Make sure to look for products that contain the multiple polyphenols present in tea as each polyphenol has unique benefits and together they create synergistic effects.

How Do the Phytonutrients in Tea Benefit Health?

In general, the catechins act throughout the body as very efficient antioxidants. The ability of these beneficial phytonutrients to detoxify free radicals and other harmful chemicals has been demonstrated beyond any doubt. In fact, the results of a study published recently in the *Journal of Agricultural and Food Chemistry* proved that the greater the catechin content of a dietary supplement, the greater its antioxidant capacity (measured in units of its "oxygen radical absorbance capacity" or "ORAC value", which is a standard measure of *in vitro* antioxidant capacity).[2]

> *"...the greater the catechin content of a dietary supplement, the greater its antioxidant capacity."*

Other research has shown that the catechins and the theaflavins all possess about the same capacity to act as antioxidants.[3] However, the total catechin content of green tea is about 2 to 3 times the total catechin plus theaflavin content of black tea (because some of the catechins are destroyed during the fermentation process).

Therefore, when consumed in equal amounts, green tea should be 2 to 3 times more effective than black tea as an antioxidant (though black tea has unique benefits all its own). This has been confirmed in experiments on hamsters that were fed diets containing very high levels of cholesterol – adding green tea to the diet of these hamsters was about twice as effective in preventing the oxidation of the cholesterol in their blood as was adding black tea.[4] Furthermore, men and women who smoke cigarettes typically exhibit a vastly accelerated rate of oxidative damage to the DNA in their bodies; when they drink 4 cups of green tea daily, they experience a large decrease in DNA free radical damage.[5,6]

Healthy Blood Pressure with Tea!

Some people and many uninformed physicians still wrongly think that caffeine intake somehow increases blood pressure. Even the U.S. Food and Drug Administration has ruled that habitual consumption of caffeine-containing foods and beverages is unrelated to blood pressure.[7] The final word should have been had by the scientists who reported recently in the *Journal of the American Medical Association* that when they studied 155,594 adult women in the United States, there was no connection between caffeine consumption and blood pressure.[8] There is no reason to fear that tea will affect this parameter of health.

Quite to the contrary – as demonstrated by a study from China.[9] Scientists found that the regular daily consumption of even only one cup of tea *enhanced* the ability to maintain blood pressure levels that are normal by 80%. The results of another study support this rather astonishing finding.[10] Tea consumption benefits the arteries and contributes to healthy blood pressure maintenance.

> "Tea consumption benefits the arteries and contributes to healthy blood pressure maintenance."

Tea Helps Keep Your Heart Healthy

Tea, especially green tea, is great for the heart. It helps keep arteries healthy, the heart pumping strong and protects cholesterol and lipids from free radical damage.

Scientists have found that tea is heart protective and the incidence of heart-related events is inversely proportional to the consumption of green tea.[11] In other words, the more green tea (or green tea catechins) you consume, the better your chances of staying heart-healthy longer.

More evidence of green tea's heart prowess comes from additional research. In one 25-year long study of the same group of elderly men in Europe, the habitual daily consumption of at least 86 mg of total catechins (equivalent to one-half cup of green tea) was found to double the chances of having optimal cardiac function with age.[12] Investigators who pooled the results of previous studies worldwide calculated that every cup of black or green tea consumed on a regular daily basis reduced the risk of heart-related events by about 4%.[13] They explained that they found a weaker effect in the overall results because in the U.S. few men drink tea. Nonetheless, these reports are consistent in concluding that healthy hearts are more common among tea drinkers.

> "Studies show again and again that those individuals consuming tea are more likely to have stronger hearts than those who consume less or none at all."

Due to the antioxidant benefits among tea drinkers, cardiac protection is increased. The catechins in green tea may directly contribute to healthy heart function by scavenging various free radical species that could be detrimental to heart tissue. Studies show again and again that those individuals consuming tea are more likely to have stronger hearts than those who consume less or none at all. For example, a study performed through Harvard University examining about 1900 men and illustrates this point well.[14] Among these men and women, those who drank one or two cups on a routine daily basis lived on average 28% longer and those who drank an average of more than two cups daily lived about 44% longer.

While it is not clear exactly what attribute of tea improved the survival and longevity of these study subjects, and a number of theories have been suggested, including the benefits of an increased antioxidant status among tea drinkers, it is clear that the benefits to the heart of tea and catechin consumption cannot be denied.

Tea Helps Keep Your Blood Flowing

There is some scientific evidence that drinking tea helps to maintain healthy blood vessel function and the delivery of oxygenated blood to the heart to keep tissues healthy. Regular tea consumption also has been reported to help blood vessels respond properly to vasodilating stimuli – in other words, the vessels expand to allow more blood to pass when more oxygenated blood is needed, especially to the heart muscle. Tea maintains circulatory function through the heart and to the peripheral tissues and organs.

The catechins in green tea not only help blood vessels respond properly to stimuli, they also help protect the interior lining of blood vessels from invasion by over-stimulated smooth muscle cells (blood vessels that can expand and contract are surrounded by smooth muscle cells that control the vessels' diameter). Catechins can thus support the pliability of vessel tissue, keeping vessels healthy and keeping them functioning as they are intended. The results of a study published recently in *Cardiovascular Research* have shown that the catechins in green tea extract prevent the secretion of enzymes by over-stimulated vascular smooth muscle cells, supporting the integrity of the lining of blood vessels and ensuring they remain healthy and undamaged, maintaining their normal structure and function. This modulatory effect of green tea catechins on blood vessel health leads to their ability to healthfully support cardiovascular function.[15]

A Healthy Skeleton Benefits from Tea – Yes, It Does!

Several decades ago, several scary articles received a great deal of publicity.[16,17] These articles attempted to show that drinking beverages containing caffeine somehow could weaken a woman's bones. — Wrong! — The real story: three more recent studies proved that the earlier articles had shown that women who drank even large amounts of beverages containing caffeine experienced reductions in bone density *only* if they also were *deficient* in calcium or vitamin D![18-20] In fact, research shows that caffeine intake has **no effect** on bones in anyone at any age.[19,20]

Drinking at least 2 cups of phytonutrient-packed black or green tea every day enhances bone health and strength. This was shown most powerfully in the 91,465 postmenopausal women who participated in the U.S. government's Women's Health Initiative study.[21] The results of this study, published in the *American Journal of Epidemiology* make it quite clear that instead of avoiding tea, women who drink at least 2 cups of tea every day can enjoy optimized bone mass throughout their bodies, and especially in parts of the vertebral spine.

Drink Tea to Keep that Belly in Line

In men and women, the degree of body fat, whether expressed as percent body fat or the ratio of waist circumference to hip circumference, tendes to decrease as green tea intake increases.[22] Green tea contributes to the maintenance of healthy body weight in several ways.

One of the least appreciated properties of green tea is its ability to limit the absorption of the fat taken in from the diet. Green tea catechins (especially EGCG) interfere with the lipase (fat-digesting) enzymes in the stomach and small intestine. The resulting incomplete digestion of fats produces some lipid droplets that are not able to enter intestinal cells and that therefore remain unabsorbed. These effects have produced significant decreases in the absorption of dietary fats by rats consuming green tea. While it is not known how effective green tea is in blocking fat absorption in humans, any interference with the normally highly efficient digestion and absorption of dietary fats could figure prominently in any effort to manage weight effectively.

In addition to decreasing the efficiency of absorption of fatty acids from the diet, green tea catechins interfere with the production of fat for storage in adipose tissue depots. Green tea leaf extract rich in EGCG, as well as purified EGCG itself, reduces the activity of fatty acid synthase, the enzyme that controls how rapidly the body produces fat for storage. This effect is consistent with a body of literature reviewed recently in the journal *Molecular Nutrition and Food Research* that shows how EGCG inhibits new fat formation ("lipogenesis") and fat storage within adipocytes.[23] Tea helps to absorb less fat from the diet and can directly interfere with the storage of fat in adipocytes, a dual mechanism for supporting healthy body weight.

The dominant green tea catechin, EGCG, also entices the body to shift some of its manner of producing energy from glucose-burning to fat-burning. There are two ways to accomplish this and EGCG seems to do both. First, if the amount of glucose available to tissues, especially the skeletal muscles, is reduced, then more fat must be metabolized to carbon dioxide and water in order to satisfy energy needs. During times when glucose is in short supply, the liver synthesizes glucose from a variety of precursors, including amino acids released by muscle cells. The first enzyme in this synthetic ("gluconeogenic") pathway, phosphoenolpyruvate carboxykinase (PEPCK), is inhibited by EGCG. Blocking this enzyme reduces the rate of formation of new glucose, requiring cells to switch to burning fat for energy.

> *"Green tea leaf extract rich in EGCG, as well as purified EGCG itself, reduces the activity of fatty acid synthase, the enzyme that controls how rapidly the body produces fat for storage."*

In an example of exquisite biochemical coordination, EGCG also stimulates the conversion of fatty acids to energy. In cell culture studies, EGCG has increased the rate of utilization of fatty acid breakdown products instead of glucose to produce energy. In a series of experiments, mice, often studied because the way they obtain energy is pretty much the same as the way humans do, have responded to the addition of catechin-rich green tea extract to a high-fat diet with less weight gain and less fat accumulation within their bodies than mice fed the same high-fat diet but not fed catechins, despite eating just as much. This phenomenon has been studied in depth. In a recent study dietary supplementation of exercising mice with tea catechins forced skeletal muscles to switch from using their glycogen reserves as energy sources to increasing their reliance on burning fats from adipose depots.[24] This "switch" is so reproducible that the researchers can predict when it will happen. The powerful phytonutrients (catechins) in green tea and green tea extract can recruit muscles to help stored fat get used up faster!

In humans, such a shift from glucose-burning to fat-burning will be seen as an increase in heat production (or thermogenesis). In a convincing demonstration of the fat-burning, thermogenic effects of green tea catechins, 24-hour heat production was measured in healthy lean to overweight young men during days in which they remained essentially at rest and consumed identical diets, no caffeine-containing foods or beverages, and either a placebo, 150 mg of caffeine alone or 150 mg of caffeine plus 270 mg of EGCG and 105 mg of other mixed catechins.[25] These investigators observed that the consumption of placebo or 150 mg of supplemental caffeine alone during a 12-hour period failed to affect the utilization of fat or glucose to supply energy. In contrast, the consumption of green tea catechins during a 12-hour period increased same-day 24-hour total energy expenditure and heat production. This increase in energy usage was caused by increased fat-burning and decreased use of glucose for fuel.

Because under the conditions of this experiment all energy expenditure was essentially "resting" energy expenditure, the catechin-induced increase in resting energy expenditure reflects enhanced thermogenesis. That is, more heat production as a "by-product" of energy production. Since increased heat production to satisfy the same energy demand means that the efficiency of energy production decreased, more stored energy needed to be "burned" – accelerating the rate at which energy stored in fat depots would become depleted. Of course, as stored fat becomes depleted, both body weight and fat depot size decrease.

The increase in fat utilization in this experiment, which was minimized by keeping the subjects in a "resting" state, could result in the loss of one pound of excess body weight in 1 to 2 months and a loss of 6 to 12 pounds in a year. Consistent with this rough prediction, overweight adults consuming 270 mg of EGCG daily for 3 months experienced an average loss of 4.6% of total body weight, with an average decrease in waist circumference of 4.5%.[26] This thermogenic effect of green tea catechins, when combined with a healthy diet and exercise, could be extremely beneficial for those looking to support weight management efforts.

Beneficial results also were obtained in a "gold standard," randomized placebo-controlled clinical trial, published recently in the *American Journal of Clinical Nutrition*.[27] In this study healthy men supplemented their diets with either 22 mg or 690 mg of total catechins daily for 12 weeks. At the end of the experiment, the men who were consuming 690 mg of total catechins daily had lost more weight, more inches off their waist, more total body fat and more abdominal fat.

What about Stress and Abdominal Fat?

A growing body of evidence indicates that in both men and women, stress and mood issues are associated with increased abdominal fat storage and a larger waistline. How is stress and belly fat connected?

Stress can increase the secretion of a hormone called cortisol. This hormone increases the rate of fat accumulation by abdominal fat cells. Even among healthy individuals, repeated episodes of stress-related cortisol secretion is implicated in increased abdominal fat.[28]

What Can Green Tea Do About It?

Green tea contains an unusual amino acid – L-theanine. This amino acid comprises up to 2.5% of the total dry weight of unfermented green tea leaves, is absorbed efficiently and can enter the brain from the blood. Within the brain, L-theanine exerts relaxing physiologic effects. In so doing, L-theanine may act to reduce perceptions of stress with possible beneficial effects on abdominal fat formation. For example, mice fed L-theanine have gained less weight and accumulated less abdominal fat.[29,30] By supporting the body's stress response, green tea and green tea extracts containing L-theanine can make important contributions to healthy weight maintenance.

Tea Helps Keep Healthy Kidneys Healthy

The kidneys are major organs involved in filtering and eliminating toxins from the body and preserving electrolytes and water. The correct performance of these functions is essential to life and critical to health and wellbeing. Green tea can help support the health of these essential organs.

"...drinking a cup of green tea at every meal can be a wise choice for individuals looking to support healthy kidney function and those interested in prevention."

Excellent scientific research vouches for the benefits your kidneys derive from tea. In a landmark study of 81,093 women who were 40 to 65 years of age when the study began in 1986 (part of the Nurses' Health Study), the investigators found that every cup of either caffeinated or decaffeinated tea consumed daily progressively enhanced the maintenance of healthy kidney function.[31] An earlier study in men had found a similar per-cup enhancement in kidney health.[32]

These findings mean that drinking a cup of green tea at every meal can be a wise choice for individuals looking to support healthy kidney function and those interested in prevention. The findings also mean that drinking 5 or 6 glasses of tea daily could be extremely beneficial. Likewise, since the benefits of tea for kidney health are probably due as much to the phytonutrients in tea as to the associated increase in water consumption, adding a dietary supplement containing the catechin equivalent of 48 ounces of tea (about 1000 mg total catechins) may yield significant benefits for healthy kidneys.

Tea Optimizes Oral Health

Wouldn't it be great if something you put into your mouth actually made it healthier? Look no further – just drink green tea. The phytonutrients in teas, especially green teas, are partially absorbed through the soft tissues of the oral cavity and "attach" to every surface, including the surfaces of the teeth. Research has shown that tea phytonutrients keep tooth surfaces clean and healthy and the tiny amount of fluoride in tea helps strengthen tooth enamel.[33] Even more impressively, a study using hamsters showed that consuming tea enhanced dental health and tooth integrity.[34] The composition of human teeth and hamster teeth is similar – so when it comes to a healthy mouth, tea consumption appears to have great potential.

There can be no doubt – for good health and healthy aging, green tea and green tea catechins are among your strongest allies.

A Word about Black Tea

Black and green teas are both derived from the same plant. Black tea is produced by fermenting tea leaves. Thus the catechins that are present in green tea are fermented to theaflavins in black tea. Theaflavins have been studied recently and found to have unique beneficial effect for cardiovascular health that go beyond the effects shown by catechins. While catechins may be more potent as antioxidants, the theaflavins support the cardiovascular system by enhancing endothelial health. A recent study found that green tea and black tea are equally effective in supporting blood vessel vasodilation and nitric oxide (NO) production.[35] Theaflavins also have potential liver-protective properties. A study found that theaflavins prevented the accumulation of lipids in the liver, suppressed the synthesis of fatty acids and stimulated fat breakdown in both laboratory and animal experiments, indicating an ability to support fat metabolism and promote liver health.[36]

Furthermore, theaflavins may help with maintaining cholesterol levels that are already in the normal range.[37] A theaflavin-enriched green tea extract was administered to 240 adult men and women in a placebo-controlled study conducted in China. The researchers found that the theaflavin-enriched green tea combination was significantly more effective than the placebo pill at supporting normal cholesterol levels when given in conjunction with a low-fat diet plan. Thus, while green tea catechins are highly beneficial, theaflavins from black tea are important compounds with cardio-protective properties.

Green Tea

- Green tea extract enhances the body's antioxidant defense systems and protects cells against free radical damage, promoting optimal cellular function.*
- Green tea extract supports a healthy cardiovascular system via its antioxidant action on lipids and its ability to support normal platelet function.*
- In cell culture and animal models, green tea reduces the formation, proliferation, and absorption of fat.*
- Green tea possesses significant thermogenic (heat-generating) properties.*
- Green tea promotes fat oxidation (fat-burning).*
- Green tea extracts may help maintain a healthy composition by reducing body fat and increasing thermogenesis and fat oxidation after eating.*
- Green tea extract has been shown to increase levels of the hormone adiponectin, which is inversely associated with percent body fat.*
- Green tea polyphenols have been shown to support the immune system, stimulating the production of several immune system cells.*

More information on these great health promoters can be obtained by visiting the Tea Council of the U.S.A. (http://www. teausa.org).

7

Phytosterols, Cholesterol and Healthy Hearts

Phytosterols are phytonutrients that occur widely throughout the plant kingdom and are present in many edible fruits, vegetables, nuts, seeds, cereals, and legumes. The most common phytosterols, **B-sitosterol, campesterol, and stigmasterol**, are *health-promoting* relatives of cholesterol – the small differences between their chemical structures and the structure of cholesterol make all the difference in the world.

Similar in form and function to cholesterol in animals and humans, phytosterols function to regulate the fluidity of cell membranes in plants.[1] Phytosterols have received a great deal of attention from researchers seeking safer means of helping people maintain healthy blood cholesterol concentrations, healthy cardiovascular systems and healthy hearts. It appears that phytosterols interfere with the intestinal recycling of the cholesterol produced by the liver, effectively reducing the availability of cholesterol to the body and may also inhibit a percentage of dietary cholesterol absorption. This is likely due to the structural similarity of these compounds with cholesterol. The most effective way of dosing plant sterols seems to be with or near a meal. While some research shows that plant sterols can be effective regardless of when they are taken, other research suggests that taking phytosterols in divided doses increases their beneficial effect.

Virtually all of the research and all of the rigorous mathematical analyses of the research that have been conducted consistently show powerful associations between phytosterol consumption (in foods or in dietary supplements) and support of healthy blood cholesterol concentrations, healthy cardiovascular systems and healthy hearts.

U.S. FDA: "Phytosterols Lower LDL-Cholesterol"

After conducting an intensive and extensive detailed review of "the totality of publicly available scientific evidence," the US Food and Drug Administration has concluded that 1) "there is significant scientific agreement to support a relationship between consumption of plant sterol esters (especially β-sitosterol, campesterol, and stigmasterol) and reduction in the risk of developing heart disease"; 2) **"plant sterol esters reduce blood total and/or LDL (the "bad" cholesterol) levels to a significant degree"**; 3) **blood HDL(the "good" cholesterol) levels are not decreased by the consumption of plant sterol esters**; and 4) these benefits can be obtained by individuals with **either elevated** blood cholesterol levels or **normal healthy** blood cholesterol levels.[2] In addition, the blood cholesterol-lowering response occurs **regardless of the composition of the rest of the diet.**

New Scientific Research: "Phytosterols Lower LDL-Cholesterol"

The conclusions reached by the US Food and Drug Administration have been echoed in the new research findings that have been published since the government's decisions. For example, a study published in the *Journal of Nutrition* showed that regardless

"It appears that phytosterols interfere with the intestinal recycling of the cholesterol produced by the liver, effectively reducing the availability of cholesterol to the body and may also inhibit a percentage of dietary cholesterol absorption."

of the nature of the diet, the cardiovascular health of men and women with blood LDL cholesterol concentrations within the "normal" range (blood LDL cholesterol concentration less than 100 mg/dL) received additional support from the addition of phytosterols to their daily diets.[3] Similar benefits were experienced in another study of men and women with initially **elevated** blood cholesterol concentrations.[4] Studies consistently have shown that phytosterols taken in the amount of 2 to 3 grams per day can reduce LDL (low density lipoprotein) cholesterol levels by about 10%.[5] In addition to their beneficial effects on blood lipid levels, phytosterols also have the ability to normalize the inflammatory response of the immune system.

A comprehensive meta-analysis published earlier this year (2009) analyzed the results of 84 clinical trials using phytosterols.[6] The authors concluded that their rigorous analysis confirmed the ability of phytosterols to significantly lower LDL cholesterol levels. The ability of phytosterols to reduce LDL concentrations was found to be dose-dependant. Again, they concluded that approximately 2 grams of phytosterols taken on a daily basis seemed to reduce LDL cholesterol by nearly 10%.

Phytosterols can be added to the diet as peanut oil, extra virgin olive oil, sesame oil, soybean oil, raw or roasted peanuts, hazelnuts, macadamia nuts, flax seed, cashews, almonds, pecans, pistachios, sunflower seeds, walnuts or as a high-quality dietary supplement.

FDA Qualified Health Claim: *Dietary supplements containing at least 400 mg of plant sterols, taken twice daily with meals for a daily total of at least 800 mg, as part of a diet low in saturated fat and cholesterol may reduce the risk of heart disease.*

8

Allicin – The Smell of Good Health

For many centuries alliums have been grown for their characteristic flavors and beautiful flowers. In addition to its esthetic and culinary attributes, the root bulb ("clove") of garlic (*Allium sativum*) has been cherished by many cultures as a powerful promoter of good health.

Sanskrit records contain evidence that garlic was being used "medicinally" about 5,000 years ago and about 4500 years ago Charak, the father of Ayurvedic medicine, claimed that garlic maintains the fluidity of blood and strengthens the heart. The 3500-year old Egyptian *Codex Ebers* touts garlic, Hippocrates and Pliny the Elder were garlicophiles, Pasteur wrote about garlic's activity in 1858 and garlic preparations were used on the battlefield in the 20th century.

Garlic and Healthy Blood Vessels

Modern research continues to affirm the health benefits that can be obtained by including raw garlic, whole garlic powders or extracts of garlic in the diet or consuming them as dietary supplements. As pointed out by the authors of a review published recently in the *Journal of Nutrition*, the evidence from studies in humans shows that the consumption of garlic supports many aspects of blood vessel health.[1] The blood vessels are the all-important corridors of the cardiovascular system. While the heart is the engine that pumps our blood, without healthy blood vessels, it can't reach the tissues where it's needed.

As an example of garlic's blood vessel-supportive prowess, the results of a human clinical trial published recently in the *Journal of Nutrition* indicated that the daily consumption of a modest amount of an extract of whole garlic cloves for 6 weeks on average doubled the ability of the brachial artery to expand in response to increased need for blood flow in healthy men and women.[2] Not only were the big blood vessels affected – the small capillaries in the skin also increased their ability to circulate fresh blood after 6 weeks of garlic consumption. Increased ability of an artery to respond to increased demand for blood flow to tissues without impacting blood pressure ("arterial compliance") and increased capacity of the small blood vessels within tissues to distribute that blood reflect a healthy cardiovascular system; this investigation provides persuasive evidence that garlic consumption is a major contributor to healthy cardiovascular function.

> "...garlic consumption is a major contributor to healthy cardiovascular function."

The results of other studies in healthy humans, also published recently in the *Journal of Nutrition* may explain how garlic can help maintain pliable arteries and open vessel channels in tissues.[3,4] In these studies investigators found that garlic has potent antioxidant properties and slows the rate of oxidation of circulating low-density lipoprotein (LDL) particles and promotes the integrity of blood vessel walls. Researchers agree that these two factors are of primary importance to maintaining excellent cardiovascular health. Keeping arteries healthy and discouraging the oxidation of lipids and fats in the blood go a long way to living a productive and heart-healthy life.

Another way garlic supports healthy blood vessels is by promoting the healthy metabolism of glucose in the blood. High blood glucose levels may adversely impact blood vessel health over time by reacting with proteins in the blood and vessels. This reaction effectively damages the protein, leading it to lose its functionality. Research published recently in the *Journal of Nutrition* shows how the bioactive compounds in garlic can prevent the formation of these sugar-protein complexes and keep your blood vessels healthy.[5] Let the proteins play their role and let blood sugar perform its function and go where it's meant to.

Where Does Allicin Come In?

A clove of garlic contains an extremely large amount of biologically active sulfur-containing phytonutrients. However, **allicin**, the most intensively studied phytonutrient associated with garlic and the source of garlic's distinctive fragrance, is not found in the clove but instead is formed when a clove is chopped, crushed, cut or chewed (breaking up the garlic cells in the clove stimulates an enzyme to produce allicin quickly). Allicin is absorbed into the human bloodstream and either exerts its benefits directly or is converted into an effective alternative compound.

Experiments in mice published recently in *Pathobiology* "connect the dots" linking allicin to garlic's vascular protective actions.[6] Dietary supplementation with pure allicin resulted in the incorporation of allicin into all lipid-containing particles produced by the intestines and liver. As the lipid particles contained allicin, they contained less cholesterol and were more resistant to oxidation. This experiment was conducted in mice that were genetically programmed to produce numerous arterial plaques as a model for atherosclerosis. The daily consumption of pure allicin drastically decreased the size of the plaques that were formed. While these mice had a genetic predisposition to a chronic condition, this dramatic illustration suggests that healthy humans with no pre-existing cardiovascular disease may benefit greatly from the consumption of garlic and allicin, as this compound promotes arterial health and wellness. The dose used in this mouse study was the equivalent of daily supplementation in humans with about 500 to 600 mg of pure allicin daily.

Enhancing Important Aspects of Cardiovascular Well-being

Humans convert some allicin into **diallyl disulfide** and **diallyl trisulfide**. These secondary phytonutrients were shown recently to impact the sequence of cholesterol synthesis in the human liver.[7] The effect of these garlic compounds in modulating healthy cholesterol metabolism and supporting antioxidant effects on blood lipids, thereby protecting their integrity and function, all add up to extremely powerful support for long-lasting healthy cardiovascular function. By impacting areas as diverse as cholesterol metabolism, arterial health, and blood sugar metabolism, garlic and its important phytonutrient constituents have become an integral part of a comprehensive plan designed to support cardiovascular wellness.

"By impacting areas as diverse as cholesterol metabolism, arterial health, and blood sugar metabolism, garlic and its important phytonutrient constituents have become an integral part of a comprehensive plan designed to support cardiovascular wellness."

Support Blood Pressure Levels that are Normal

It turns out that garlic and various garlic extracts may have additional direct cardiovascular benefits in humans. A comprehensive review of the literature was carried out and published in 2008. The authors of this meta-analysis reviewed papers in the literature dealing with the blood-pressure regulating properties of garlic in humans and found that the intake of garlic in foods and supplements contributes to the maintenance of blood pressure levels that are considered healthy in humans.[8] The researchers concluded that the blood-pressure regulating compound in garlic is allicin and that garlic's hydrogen sulfide production is also a contributory factor. A second group of researchers also conducted an independent review of the studies associating the intake of garlic supplements with blood pressure effects.[9] In their review, they also concluded that garlic supplements had an ability to support the maintenance of blood pressure levels that are already in the normal range.

The consensus is that garlic intake supports healthy blood pressure, just another of the many reasons to consider adding garlic to your daily nutritional regimen.

Support the Body's Stress Response and Increase Energy

Research into the energy-enhancing and stress-supportive effects of garlic has yielded a number of mechanisms that begin to explain the tonifying ability of this ancient food. Scientists believe that the ability of garlic to enhance peripheral circulation, its antioxidant effects that protect the brain and peripheral tissues, its ability to support and promote a healthy immune defense, and simply its nutritional value lend it to be well-suited for these benefits. Garlic is a good source of numerous essential vitamins and minerals. The attributes of its various constituents play a vital role in the tonic abilities of this herb. However, researchers feel the fact that the constituents of whole garlic exert synergistic effects in the presence of one another are a more likely explanation of it benefits. Several animal experiments and some human experiments have shown stress-relieving and endurance-enhancing abilities of this herb.[10] Whatever the reasons may be, what was true in ancient times remains so now - garlic is a mental and physical rejuvenator.

> *"...what was true in ancient times remains so now - garlic is a mental and physical rejuvenator."*

And If that's Not Enough...

The benefits of allicin are not limited to the cardiovascular system. Daily dietary supplementation with allicin can increase the activity of the human "immunosurveillance system" – that is, the vigilance of the immune system to seek out and repair damaged cells.[11,12] This innate "Homeland Security Force" serves to preserve and protect the "normality" of the complex internal cellular network that is your body. Keeping your immunosurveillance set to "high alert" and on constant patrol supports and defends the healthy function of every organ and tissue.

Allicin

- Allicin, found in garlic, supports healthy circulation.*
- Allicin supports cardiovascular health by helping to maintain healthy blood vessel elasticity.*
- Allicin helps maintain normal blood vessel tone by supporting production of nitric oxide, a key regulator of blood vessel function.*
- Allicin supports normal contraction and relaxation of blood vessels by activating nitric oxide synthase, a key enzyme that regulates production of nitric oxide.*
- Allicin helps maintain cholesterol levels already within the normal range.*
- Allicin helps maintain blood lipid levels already within the normal range.*
- Allicin helps maintain the ability of LDL to resist oxidation by free radicals.*
- Allicin helps the body defend itself against free radicals.*
- Allicin shows promise as a dietary ingredient that can help preserve cardiovascular function.*
- Allicin may help maintain the body's production of antioxidant enzymes.*

9

CoQ10 – The Vital Link Between Energy and Your Heart

CoQ$_{10}$ – Pivotal Player in Cellular Energy Production

Coenzyme Q$_{10}$ (CoQ$_{10}$) is a ubiquitous compound (hence the proper name, ubiquinone) that occurs in every cell in the body. The main function of CoQ$_{10}$ is to maintain a rapid rate of conversion of oxygen (O$_2$) to water (H$_2$O) in the mitochondria of a cell. In the process, the free electrons produced during the chemical conversion of sugars and fats into chemical energy are captured and transferred (along with protons; H$^+$) to oxygen molecules. The energy released in reducing oxygen (O$_2$) to water (H$_2$O) is harnessed to produce ATP, the carrier of chemical energy from the mitochondria to the rest of the cell.

CoQ$_{10}$ is absolutely required in order for the free electrons to reach the oxygen within a cell. In fact, CoQ$_{10}$ is the lynchpin in the entire "electron transport chain," linking the molecules that shuttle the free electrons through the cell to the special proteins ("cytochromes") that deliver the electrons directly to O$_2$ molecules.

Because CoQ_{10} plays such a central role in hooking up electrons and oxygen, the amount of CoQ_{10} available determines the rate of energy production by a cell – even if there are plenty of oxygen and electrons "in waiting." Humans can synthesize CoQ_{10} endogenously and therefore it is not considered a vitamin. However, research shows that CoQ_{10} levels decline with age and with the use of certain medications. Hence, supplementation of CoQ_{10} is needed to replenish levels. CoQ_{10} availability in the cells' mitochondria is a major determinant of energy production and, therefore, the speed and power of contraction in heart muscle cells ("cardiomyocytes") and, in fact, in all muscles.[1]

CoQ_{10}, Heart Muscle Energetics and Cardiac Contraction

A systematic review published recently determined that supplementation with CoQ_{10} enhanced the strength of cardiac contractions in men and women by an average of one-third.[3] This relatively enormous increase in cardiac power delivered substantially more oxygenated blood throughout the body. These conclusions mirrored the findings of a study that were published in the *European Heart Journal* after that analysis was complete. This human clinical trial confirmed the beneficial effects of CoQ_{10} supplementation on human heart muscle while also showing that these benefits were accompanied by a large increase in exercise capacity – proof that the increase in cardiac power was beneficial to the entire body.[4]

Clearly, CoQ_{10} is a powerful ally in maintaining efficient cardiac mechanics and function.

> "A systematic review published recently determined that supplementation with CoQ10 enhanced the strength of cardiac contractions in men and women by an average of one-third."

CoQ$_{10}$ Deficiency and "Cellular Exhaustion"

Individuals that have a deficiency of CoQ10 are inefficient in converting O_2 to H_2O and, therefore, are unable to generate adequate cellular energy. They suffer the consequences of "cellular exhaustion", which may lead to the impairment of several normal physiological functions. These effects can be seen in the functioning of organs such as the brain, digestive tract, eyes and heart, and can also lead to decreases in energy levels and exercise capacity. As shown recently in the *Archives of Neurology* dietary supplementation with CoQ$_{10}$ can restore the rate of mitochondrial respiration, muscle strength, coordination and exercise tolerance[5], which highlights the ability of CoQ10 to support the healthy function of several systems by promoting cellular health.

CoQ$_{10}$, Endurance and "Energy"

It is clear that all muscles – heart, legs, arms, chest – benefit from ample supplies of CoQ$_{10}$. The efficiency of muscular work, the amount of energy expended during work and the ability to harness that energy in productive and enjoyable activities all depend on the presence of adequate amounts of CoQ$_{10}$. As shown by studies such as those published in the *European Heart Journal*[4] and the *Archives of Neurology*[5], increasing the supply of CoQ$_{10}$ that is available to all muscles is invaluable in supporting their efforts to work harder, faster and longer. CoQ$_{10}$ supports both aspects of activity – intensity and duration. By increasing the maximum work intensity that can be achieved, CoQ$_{10}$ may help routine daily life seem to be easier and require less effort. By increasing the length of time that activities can be enjoyed, ensuring adequate CoQ$_{10}$ levels can help postpone feelings of tiredness.

Although CoQ$_{10}$ will not give you "energy" – that requires a healthy diet – CoQ$_{10}$ will help you use your energy more effectively – making you feel more energetic, active and healthy.

CoQ$_{10}$ as a Buffer against Toxic Cellular Acidity

As an integral component of cellular membranes, CoQ$_{10}$ also facilitates the exchange of sodium ions (Na$^+$) for protons (H$^+$) across the plasma membrane of all cells. As a potent antioxidant nutrient, CoQ$_{10}$ molecules residing within the cell membrane can "grab" free electrons from within the cell and pass them along to electron acceptor molecules outside the cell, while the CoQ$_{10}$ itself remains snuggly within the membrane. This exchange prevents the inside of the cell from becoming too acidic – a condition that could lead to cellular damage. The free radical scavenging activity of CoQ10 makes it an extremely useful cellular protectant.

CoQ$_{10}$ and Heart Muscle Longevity

The role of CoQ10 as a cellular protectant is displayed in a more direct fashion in heart cells. CoQ$_{10}$ plays an important part in supporting the maintenance of cardiac tissue integrity and function. A relatively recently explored hypothesis suggests that CoQ$_{10}$ can slow the rate of normal age-related loss of cardiomyocytes, preserving more fully functional cells for longer. Within the mitochondria of all mammalian cells, including the heart muscle (the "myocardium"), are channels ("permeability transition pores") that span the inner and outer mitochondrial membranes (every mitochondrion has a double wrapping of membrane material surrounding it and separating it from the rest of the cell). When open, these channels allow materials to pass from the cell into the mitochondrion and *vice versa*. Normally, traffic between the cell and the mitochondrion is strictly controlled.

However, if too many of these channels open at once, abnormal movements of sodium and calcium ions break down the physical integrity of the mitochondrial membrane, and the membrane will be destroyed by the cell.[6] If too many mitochondria within the same cell become damaged and are destroyed, the cell will die.

The channels can be opened "accidentally" by "stray" free electrons that have escaped from the special proteins that should be transporting them toward oxygen. Escape is less likely when sufficient CoQ_{10} is available to restrain these electrons. As shown by the results of a study published recently in the *Journal of Gerontology* and the results of previous studies, the more CoQ_{10} in the mitochondria, the fewer channels that are opened "accidentally" and the less likely the cell will be to die.[7]

CoQ_{10} – Super Antioxidant

We touched on some of the antioxidant effects of CoQ10 earlier. Research suggests that CoQ10 has superior antioxidant properties and works in a broad range of environments. It is a powerful and effective protector of lipids, low-density lipoproteins, proteins and DNA from oxidation. For example, increasing the CoQ_{10} content of rat heart muscle cells and brain neurons through the diet reduces the ability of free electrons to cause oxidative damage to those cells. A study published recently in *Neurobiology of Disease* has shown that CoQ10 also protects human neurons.[8] This protective property of CoQ_{10} provides firm scientific evidence that dietary supplementation with this nutrient can increase the resistance of mitochondrial membranes, proteins and DNA to oxidative damage, especially in the tissues that are the most sensitive to such damage.[9]

CoQ_{10} – Preserver of Mitochondrial Health and Function

The "mitochondrial theory of aging" postulates that the accumulation of free radical-induced damage to mitochondrial DNA in mature cells (such as cardiomyocytes) eventually results in the production of abnormal mitochondrial proteins.[9] These abnormal proteins cannot sequester and restrain free electrons as well as they should and more electrons escape to cause even more oxidative damage in an escalating vicious cycle.

In addition, because fewer free electrons reach oxygen molecules, the cell cannot produce a normal amount of energy.[9]

If this theory is correct, then maintaining a high level of cellular and mitochondrial CoQ_{10} through dietary supplementation can sustain a high degree of efficient energy metabolism within mitochondria and can make a fundamental contribution to maximal cellular health and function. As shown in recently published studies CoQ_{10} protects mitochondria from "runaway" free electrons – and nowhere will this contribution be as appreciated as within the human heart.[10,11]

As an added antioxidant benefit, CoQ_{10} also spares vitamin C and vitamin E. As these vitamins perform their antioxidant functions and become oxidized themselves, they are likely to be excreted in the urine – which means that each such "lost" vitamin C or vitamin E molecule must be replaced through the diet or through supplementation. Fortunately, CoQ_{10} is able to receive their free electrons, effectively recycling these nutrients for use as antioxidants and allowing them to continue protecting the body from oxidative damage.[12,13] The free electron-carrying CoQ_{10} molecule then is able to transfer the electron to other antioxidant molecules, retaining the sequestration of the electron while regenerating itself.[12]

Control Your Cholesterol – and Just Your Cholesterol!

The effectiveness of the HMG-CoA reductase inhibitor drugs, the so-called "statins," in lowering serum cholesterol concentration cannot be denied. However, CoQ10 production and cholesterol synthesis share the same biochemical pathway. As could be predicted from these pathways in the liver effectively blocking cholesterol production can also lead to blocking CoQ_{10} production. Numerous studies have proven this to be the case.[14,15]

The results of this drug-induced mild CoQ_{10} deficiency is not without harm – it is associated with damage to hard-working muscles. These potentially detrimental effects have been reported in several journals.[16,17] In terms of the side effects of statin therapy, published studies have found fundamental derangements in muscle cell metabolism with exposure to statins.[18] Several recent reports indicate that these drugs impact the nerves that communicate with muscles in addition to affecting the mitochondria of all muscles, including the heart muscle.[19,20] Depleted levels of CoQ10 could play a major role in these side effects of statin drugs.

The good news – dietary supplementation with CoQ_{10} may help overcome the potential interference of statin drugs with CoQ_{10} metabolism.[21] And CoQ_{10} is very safe – amounts of up to 3000 mg daily are considered safe.[22]

Thus, if you choose to use cholesterol-lowering medication to protect your heart and circulatory system, don't be counter-productive. *Really* protect yourself – supplement with CoQ_{10} to replenish what you lose with the use of statin drugs. Add this vital nutrient to your Healthy Heart program.

> *"The good news – dietary supplementation with CoQ10 may help overcome the potential interference of statin drugs with CoQ10 metabolism."*

CoQ_{10} Softgels Better than Tablets

Dietary supplements are available that deliver CoQ_{10} in several different ways. The most common means are via tablets, hard-shell powder-filled capsules or soft-shelled capsules that enclose CoQ_{10} in a suspension of oil. Human research has shown that CoQ_{10} is absorbed most efficiently and rapidly when consumed suspended within a soft-shelled capsule.[23] Since CoQ10 is a fat-soluble nutrient, taking it in an oil matrix or with a meal containing fat is highly beneficial. Thus, when considering supplemental forms of CoQ_{10} "softgels" are an excellent choice.

Ubiquinone or Ubiquinol?

A new form of CoQ10 has come on the market in recent years. This form is the reduced form of CoQ10 known as ubiquinol.

Most CoQ10 on the market is in the oxidized ubiquinone form. While this form is adequate for most individuals for dietary supplement purposes, it may not be effective for some. When ubiquinone CoQ10 is taken in by the body, it is converted to the reduced form, ubiquinol. However, as we age our bodies lose the ability to convert rapidly between the two forms. Since ubiquinol is the reduced form, it more readily is able to scavenge free radicals and may be more effective in people over 40 or 45 years of age. Another benefit of using the ubiquinol form is that the dosage needed can be reduced since ubiquinol is already the active form of CoQ10.

Until recently, the stability of ubiquinol in capsule form was questionable and this made it difficult to manufacture an effective form of this nutrient. However, technological advancements have allowed for the manufacture of stable ubiquinol for supplemental purposes. The choice is yours. Both forms are effective and the original ubiquinone form of CoQ10 (the majority of CoQ10 on the market) is the one with the best science at this point. Most studies have used the original ubiquinone form. However, for some people, the reduced form, ubiquinol, may be more beneficial.

CoQ10

- Helps prevent negative effects of aging. CoQ10 levels tend to decrease with age, thus supplementing with this nutrient can help support energy production and protect the cells of the heart, brain and other organs during the normal aging process. *
- CoQ10 is a fat-soluble antioxidant that can help prevent oxidative damage to cells, tissues and organs, thus protecting the body from pro-oxidative conditions such as stress and environmental pollution. CoQ10 both acts as an antioxidant itself as well as helps to regenerate other known antioxidants such as vitamins C and E. *

Heart and Cardiovascular Support

- The heart is the hardest working muscle in the body. Because of its high energy requirements, the heart needs CoQ10 at all times.*
- Numerous clinical studies have demonstrated CoQ10's significant ability to promote heart function with oral administration.*
- Many statin drugs, which are commonly used to lower cholesterol levels, are known to deplete CoQ10. CoQ Max 100 Super Formula provides supplemental CoQ10 to meet losses caused by statin drug therapy.*
- Supports a healthy cardiovascular system through antioxidant activity.*
- As an antioxidant, CoQ10 may help prevent the free radical induced oxidation of fats stored in our bodies.*
- CoQ10 may help maintain healthy blood pressure levels that are already in the normal range.*
- CoQ10 may help maintain normal vascular tone.*
- CoQ10 may help support normal blood vessel relaxation.*

Helps Maintain Healthy Energy Production

- CoQ10 works at the cellular level to produce energy for metabolism in the form of ATP.*
- CoQ10 is a necessary component in the energy producing systems known as the "Krebs cycle" and the "electron transport chain" in which cells use sugar and oxygen to make energy (in the form of ATP). *
- Without an adequate supply of CoQ10, cells can become energy-deficient, slowing down a number of critical cellular processes.*
- As an antioxidant, CoQ10 may support normal oxygen delivery to cells, aiding in healthy cellular metabolism.*
- Muscle cells are some of the most active cells in the body, demanding a large supply of energy in the form of ATP.

CoQ10 plays a critical role in the production of ATP, thus supporting the proper function of the musculoskeletal system.*

Brain Support/ Neuro-Protection

- Studies have shown that CoQ10's potent free radical scavenging properties extend to brain tissue, where CoQ10 may protect neurons from the ravages of oxidative damage.*
- As a fat-soluble antioxidant, CoQ10 can help prevent oxidative damage to neuronal cell membranes and aid in proper communication between neurons.*
- CoQ10's antioxidant properties can also help protect neurons during times of stress.*

Immune Function Support

- Immune cells need large amounts of energy to carry out their defensive functions. CoQ10 is required for this energy to be available.*
- Research on animals has shown that CoQ10 enhances immune functions such as the activity of phagocytes and antibody production.*

10

Vitamins and Minerals – Helping Hands of Health

The vitamins and essential minerals are just that – essential. They must be part of the diet every day, day after day, year after year. Long-term failure to include enough of even one vitamin or essential mineral from the diet will cause disease, cell death and tissue degeneration. Eventually, the entire body will begin to die. Obviously, this is not a scenario consistent with the goal of Healthy Aging, as deficiencies of essential minerals and vitamins are the unhealthiest way to age. In the paradigm of healthy aging, ensuring adequate intakes of these essentials is the first step. Without this essential foundation, the other pillars of healthy aging crumble fast.

By now, in this enlightened, affluent, highly-educated era, it would seem reasonable to expect that no one in the US could possibly suffer from a deficiency of a vitamin or essential mineral. Or so the US government and the American Medical Association may have you believe. Unfortunately, it just isn't so.

According to US government data, over 90% of all adult Americans do not consume enough calcium every day to satisfy the current government-sanctioned (that is, minimal) dietary standards. The same holds true for magnesium and vitamin E.

Another 75% of all US adults are deficient in copper or zinc; half are deficient in vitamin C, vitamin D or chromium; and between 10% and 15% are deficient in one or more of the B-vitamins. Amazingly, even in the face of the current epidemic of obesity, widespread nutritional deficiencies are rampant in the US. We're eating more than ever in the history of human existence. Yet, what we're eating more of is empty calories. Processed foods are a high percentage of the Standard American Diet (So SAD!) and these foods are devoid of many essential vitamins and minerals. So while we're eating more, we're not consuming enough of the essentials.

You might ask, "So what? I don't feel unhealthy." It's not like we have problems with:

> *"According to US government data, over 90% of all adult Americans do not consume enough calcium every day to satisfy the current government-sanctioned (that is, minimal) dietary standards."*

GUM HEALTH (vitamin C and magnesium);

HAIR HEALTH and rough skin (B-vitamins);

PROSTATE HEALTH (vitamin D, vitamin E, selenium and zinc);

HEALTHY BLOOD SUGAR (chromium, magnesium and vanadium);

BONE HEALTH (calcium, magnesium, boron, vitamin D, vitamin C, vitamin E, vitamin K);

MEMORY ISSUES (folate/folic acid, thiamin, choline, vitamin E, selenium);

HEART HEALTH (selenium, calcium, magnesium, vitamin C, vitamin E and vitamin D);

PERIODONTAL HEALTH (calcium, magnesium, vitamin C and vitamin D);

WEAK IMMUNE SYSTEMS (selenium, zinc, vitamin C and vitamin D); or

FEELING TIRED (B-vitamins and magnesium),

These issues are so prevalent in our population that it's easy not to be concerned about them. The more one thinks about them, though, the more one realizes the problems they can lead to. The irony of it all is that these areas can all be supported simply by ensuring adequate intakes of essential vitamins and minerals.

In addition to the prevention of the classically recognized nutritional deficiency diseases, healthy intakes of vitamins and minerals can do the body a world of good. A few stellar examples should make the point.

> *"Sufficient antioxidants in the body that quench potentially harmful free radicals promote health and longevity."*

Vitamins, Minerals and Longevity

—Antioxidant Vitamins and Minerals

The antioxidant mineral, **selenium,** and antioxidant **carotenoids** (especially -carotene, **lutein, lycopene, zeaxanthin** and **B-cryptoxanthin**) have been shown to increase your chances of living longer. The results of a study published recently in the *Journal of Nutrition* **clearly showed just that – women with the most selenium and carotenoids in their bodies tended to live the longest.**[1] And since, in this respect at least, men and women are not different, the same conclusion can be applied to men. Increasingly, research is showing that sufficient antioxidants in the body that quench potentially harmful free radicals promote health and longevity.

Vitamins, Minerals and the Brain

— Folate

Folate sufficiency has long been associated with protection of mental ability and particularly so in older adults. The link between folate and brain health was confirmed by the results of a "gold standard" randomized, placebo-controlled human clinical trial, reported very recently in the prestigious medical journal *Lancet*.[2] **During the 3 years of this study, men and women who were over 50 years old consumed either a placebo tablet or 800 mcg of folic acid daily (folic acid is a commonly used form of folate in dietary supplements).** After 3 years, the subjects who had been supplementing their diets with folic acid had experienced greater memory and recall skills, quickness of thought and ability to react physically to a visual stimulus.

In these same subjects, as reported separately in the *Annals of Internal Medicine* this amount of supplemental folic acid was shown to support hearing function and prevent normal decline of hearing with age.[3] In addition, after 3 years of folic acid supplementation, all of the supplemented subjects who had higher levels of homocysteine at the beginning of the study, but none of the initially hyperhomocysteinemic "placebo" subjects, had normalized their blood homocysteine concentrations. What is surprising is that in spite of massive governmental efforts to convince adults to consume 400 mcg of folic acid daily, none of the subjects in this study were consuming more than 250 mcg daily before the study began.

These experimental findings echo an avalanche of observational studies published recently in the *American Journal of Clinical Nutrition*. **For example, the greater the dietary intake of folate by men and women over the age of 69, the better their language skills (word recognition and use), memory recall, ability to copy simple drawings (a test of visual-motor integration) and ability to think abstractly.**[4]

Similarly, the abilities of Chinese men and women over 55 years old to learn and use new words and to remember facts were greater the more folate and folic acid they consumed on a daily.[5] In another study the diet and cognitive abilities of men over 50 years old and participating in the Veterans' Affairs Normative Aging Study were measured. Compared to the men who were consuming the current RDA for folate, those men consuming at least 25% more folate exhibited better visual-motor integration and were better able to remember the meanings of words. [6]

Yet another study reported that the overall cognitive functioning ability of 85-year old men and women improved as daily folate intake increased.[7] Still more research reported that in men and women over the age of 65, as dietary folate intake increased, so also did verbal learning ability, problem-solving ability and the speed of mental information processing.[8] Finally, the onset of clinically important age-related loss of overall cognitive function was delayed in men and women with the greatest dietary intakes of folate[9], indicating the memory-supportive ability of this critical vitamin.

All of these benefits occurred whether folate was consumed as foods or as supplements in the form of folic acid.

Clearly, folate and folic acid are staunch supporters of brain health – especially healthy brain aging.

—*Thiamin*

The importance of the B-vitamins during human fetal development cannot be overemphasized. Certainly, the prevention of neural tube defects with folate is "proof of principle" – contrary to some old misconceptions among obstetricians, maternal nutrition has a profound impact on even the earliest stages of the formation and development of the human mind. As shown most recently in work published in *Brain Research* poor **thiamin** status during pregnancy (which affects between 1 in 5 and 1 in 10 of all human embryos) stunts the size of the newborn brain by effectively shortening the lives of the first generations of brain cells.[10]

—*Choline*

Choline is a B-vitamin-like nutrient that is required for the synthesis of essential components of nerve and brain cell membranes. In humans, the rate of synthesis of these components is governed by the availability of choline in the brain, which itself is determined by dietary choline intake. **When incoming supplies of choline are inadequate, existing neuronal cell membranes**

will be "cannibalized" for their choline – obviously a losing proposition in the long run. In contrast, dietary supplementation with choline prevents such avoidable loss of brain cell integrity.

—Vitamin E

Because **vitamin E** is a strong antioxidant, especially in tissues with large ratios of cell membranes to total cell volume (such as the brain), it has long been thought that this vitamin must play an important, health-sustaining role in protecting brain membrane lipids from oxidation. Such a role has been confirmed by the research results that have been published very recently in the Chinese medical journal, *Acta Biochimica et Biophysica Sinica*.[11] **When human brain cells were grown in the laboratory and were exposed to -amyloid plaques, the cells suffered widespread oxidative damage. However, when vitamin E also was present, the cells were protected from such damage.** These findings confirm that vitamin E is a strong antioxidant protector within the human brain and promotes healthy brain structure.

—Selenium

The usefulness of any nutrient to the brain depends on the ability of that nutrient to reach and enter the brain. Several systems, together called the "blood-brain barrier," work to regulate the nature and amount of both desirable and undesirable compounds and nutrients that can gain access to the human brain. For example, **selenium** is a very beneficial antioxidant for the central nervous system, once it passes through the blood-brain barrier. However, as shown in research on live mice published recently in the *Journal of Biological Chemistry* the ability of selenium to reach the brain is hindered unless the amount of selenium in the blood is sufficient to activate the carrier proteins that transfer selenium from the blood into the brain.[12] **In other words, if dietary selenium is inadequate, the brain can become effectively "selenium starved."** Of course, selenium has immense usefulness as an antioxidant in other tissues. Hence, the body requires selenium for other needs, ultimately potentially depriving the brain when levels are inadequate.

Vitamins, Minerals and the Cardiovascular System

—*Vitamin C; Vitamin E*

Vitamin C and **vitamin E** protect lipids from oxidation in the blood and stimulate the immune system to remove from the circulation any cholesterol-containing particles that have become oxidized. These actions both protect the health of the cardiovascular system and promote the health of blood vessels in the body.

—*Calcium*

Maintaining the proper degree of sensitivity to stimuli that allows blood vessels to swell or constrict according to the body's needs is an unappreciated function of the **calcium** that is circulating in your bloodstream. If there is not enough calcium available, blood vessels become stiff and tend to lose their ability to relax – a situation that causes the blood pressure to remain elevated even when the body does not need the extra pressure to distribute blood where it's needed. In recognition of the importance of calcium supply to a healthy cardiovascular system, on October 12, 2005, the U.S. Food and Drug Administration announced that "Some scientific evidence suggests that calcium supplements may reduce the risk of hypertension." Furthermore, as a key contributor to the modulatory function of blood vessel relaxation, calcium supplementation may support

> *"Maintaining the proper degree of sensitivity to stimuli that allows blood vessels to swell or constrict according to the body's needs is an unappreciated function of the calcium that is circulating in your bloodstream."*

the body's ability to maintain blood pressure in individuals whose pressures are already in the normal range.

—Magnesium

The heart muscle is exquisitely sensitive to all aspects of its environment, including the amount of magnesium available to it. Adequate magnesium can translate into increased heart health, with longevity benefits. As shown in research published recently in the *Canadian Journal of Physiology and Pharmacology*, magnesium reduces the toxicity of the oxidative substances that are produced during normal cardiac contractions.[13] Magnesium also acts to stabilize the electrical excitability of the heart muscle, promotes normal cardiac rhythms and increases the efficiency of energy use by the myocardium. Research also suggests that daily magnesium intakes of 300 mg also relax skeletal muscles and foster restful sleep in individuals prone to leg cramps at night.

In addition to actions within the heart itself, magnesium also helps maintain the patency of blood vessels, with positive effects on the maintenance of blood pressure levels that are already normal. And because magnesium facilitates the regulation of cholesterol synthesis and metabolism, adequate magnesium levels may promote serum LDL-cholesterol and HDL-cholesterol concentrations that are already in the normal range, as shown most recently in several published research studies.[14,15]

> "Magnesium also acts to stabilize the electrical excitability of the heart muscle, promotes normal cardiac rhythms and increases the efficiency of energy use by the myocardium."

The beneficial longevity-enhancing effects of magnesium on the heart and cardiovascular system are well documented. This has been demonstrated clearly in the results of a 10-year study of over 14,000 adult men published recently in *Environmental Health Perspectives*.[16] **The investigators found that as daily magnesium intake increased, the health of the heart**

also increased, confirming a large body of existing evidence. In fact, several studies suggest that a daily intake of at least 400 mg of magnesium powerfully supports healthy cardiovascular function with age.

The evidence is in – and provides ample justification (and motivation) for adding magnesium to the list of nutrients that promote heart health and longevity.

Vitamins, Minerals and the Skeleton

—Calcium

Of course, calcium is the major structural component supporting skeletal health. Increasing calcium intake (through foods or dietary supplements) increases bone integrity and provides a structure that is much less likely to fail (that is, break). This biological truism has been confirmed over and over by the results of "gold standard" randomized placebo-controlled clinical trials. As discussed in a detailed review published recently in the *Brazilian Archives of Endocrinology and Metabolism*, dietary supplementation with calcium prevents bone fractures – even in adults who already had suffered osteoporotic fractures (and therefore had very weak bones) before adding sufficient calcium to their diets.[17]

The U.S. Food and Drug Administration has recognized the relationship between good calcium nutrition and bone health by stating that "Adequate calcium throughout life, as part of a well-balanced diet, may reduce the risk of osteoporosis."

—Vitamin D

Although other nutrients are vital components of a strong skeletal structure, it is increasingly clear that **vitamin D** is the manager that orchestrates skeletal health. A deluge of new information emphasizes the importance of vitamin D – a degree of importance even greater than has been thought before. In fact, the results of the Women's Health Initiative published recently in the *New England Journal of Medicine* proved that the need for vitamin D is much greater than previously believed.[18] Fortunately, daily supplementation with enough vitamin D can be quite effective in promoting a strong long-lived skeleton.[19] The question arises as to how much is enough? The independent Vitamin D Council (www.vitamindcouncil.com) suggests that otherwise healthy adults who get some sunshine every day should consume 1000 IU of vitamin D daily – if moderate sun exposure is not possible, 2000 IU would be preferable.

> *"...the need for Vitamin D is much greater than previously believed."*

These levels are very safe, despite the fact that they are much higher than was believed to be adequate just a few years ago. However, these levels may not be high enough for everyone. Individuals should check with their doctors about being tested for blood levels of vitamin D (a relatively easy test to conduct). If levels are low, an appropriate regimen should be instituted to raise vitamin D levels.

—Magnesium

The third member of the major bone-building trio is magnesium. While calcium deficiency predisposes both men and women to thin bones and spontaneous fractures, this mineral is just as important as it promotes healthy mineral retention by bone tissue. Much more importantly, as shown in research results published recently in the *Journal of the American Geriatric Society* and the *Journal of Clinical Endocrinology and Metabolism* the density and strength of every bone in the human body is proportional to the intake of magnesium.[20,21]

—Vitamin C

While most emphasis is placed on the mineral components of bone tissue, without **vitamin C** to band together the collagen fibers that actually form bones, there would be no guide to the placement of minerals and bone tissue would be fragmented and without mechanical strength. **As vitamin C is required for collagen synthesis, bone strength is dependent on vitamin C supply.**[22]

Strong bones require healthy joints in order for the skeleton to do more than simply support your weight against the pull of gravity. Modern research has shown that adequate consumption of vitamin C helps sustain healthy joints and promote their continued function.[23,24]

—Vitamin E

The connection between maintaining oxidant/antioxidant balance and continuing skeletal health is only now being appreciated. This connection is underscored by the recent discovery that antioxidant capacity, especially **vitamin E** status, can be severely compromised in adults with joint issues.[25] Enhancing antioxidant defense systems may indeed be a key factor in sustaining healthy joint and skeletal function as antioxidants can prevent damage to join tissue from free radicals.

—Boron

Although the trace mineral **boron** is found within bone, its function there is not yet entirely clear. However, it is known that rats fed a boron-free diet develop weak bones. In fact, boron supplementation in rats and chicks has been found to increase bone strength. Furthermore, boron influences the metabolism of several metabolic enzymes in various ways as well as the metabolism of steroid hormones and nutrients including vitamin D, calcium and magnesium.[26]

—Vitamin K

Vitamin K is required for the production of the non-collagen proteins in bone. This means that, because vitamin K helps determine the amount of non-mineral bone tissue that is available to be mineralized, human bone mineral density is proportional to vitamin K intake. The findings of an extensive analysis of published research have determined that poor vitamin K status dramatically increases the chances of bone fractures.[27] A new concept in human nutrition is that because humans rely on gut bacteria to produce vitamin K from dietary fiber, the typical low-vegetable, low-fiber diet may be causing a form of undiagnosed vitamin K deficiency, manifested as impaired bone health. Of course, vitamin K is essential for other systems as well, an important one being the cardiovascular system. The preferred form of vitamin K seems to be vitamin K2, menaquinone, which is free of toxicity and has been shown to have the best bone-supportive and cardiovascular benefits. The optimal form of vitamin K2 is known as MK-7 and is derived from a fermented Asian soy food known as natto.

Vitamins, Minerals and the Prostate Gland

—Selenium

Selenium is a potent supporter of prostate health. According to scientists who published the results of a detailed analysis of the scientific evidence **dietary supplementation with 100 mcg of selenium every day can contribute substantially to the long-term health and healthy function of a man's prostate.**[28] It seems that the way in which selenium works is that it "seeks out" the cells of the prostate and, by helping to maintain a healthy oxidant/antioxidant balance, promotes sustained health of these all-important cells.[29]

> "In promoting prostate health, the US Food and Drug Administration announced on February 21, 2003, that "Selenium may reduce the risk of certain cancers."

In fact, in promoting prostate health, the US Food and Drug Administration announced on February 21, 2003, that "Selenium may reduce the risk of certain cancers. Some scientific evidence suggests that consumption of selenium may reduce the risk of certain forms of cancer" and "Selenium may produce anticarcinogenic effects in the body. Some scientific evidence suggests that consumption of selenium may produce anticarcinogenic effects in the body." These statements highlight the importance of receiving an adequate supply of this nutrient.

—Vitamin E

While selenium powerfully protects the inner workings of prostate cells, their cell membranes also need defense against oxidative invasion. This is where **vitamin E** fits in. Recent scientific evidence illustrates the important role of vitamin E in maintaining prostate health by promoting its antioxidant effects on prostate cells.[30,31]

—Zinc

Prostate health isn't just a matter of antioxidants. It also depends on proper metabolic control of energy processing within the gland. Even early loss of a small part of regulatory control can decrease prostate health. Although the regulation of energy processing is a complex process in any cell, a few quirks in the way prostate cells handle this challenge have placed the mineral, **zinc**, in a pivotal position. Recently published research illustrates the role of zinc in prostate function and highlights **the special needs of the prostate for zinc.**[32] **The prostate needs zinc for health – so all men need zinc for prostate health.**

Vitamins, Minerals and Normal Blood Glucose Regulation

—Chromium

Chromium is an absolutely vital cofactor that allows insulin to effectively stimulate the transfer of glucose from the blood into cells. The functions of chromium are so important that the

US Food and Drug Administration has reviewed the evidence on chromium picolinate and allowed a qualified health claim on products containing this form of chromium stating that chromium picolinate may reduce the risk of insulin resistance and therefore, may possibly reduce the risk of type 2 (adult-onset) diabetes.

—Magnesium

In addition to chromium, adequate **magnesium** intake is required for maintenance of stable blood sugar levels. As dietary magnesium intake goes up, the efficiency of glucose storage by muscle cells increases. This principle was demonstrated in the results of a study published recently in which elevated magnesium status was associated with healthy blood sugar control in children.[33] Of course, the healthier our blood sugar management is, the healthier we will be. The link between healthy magnesium nutrition and healthy blood glucose regulation is underscored by the results of analyses of the data obtained from the 85,060 female nurses participating in the Nurses' Health Study, the 39,345 women participating in the Women's Health Study and the 42,872 men participating in the Health Professionals Follow-Up Study – **those individuals who regularly consumed at least 400 mg of magnesium daily had significantly better blood sugar regulation in conjunction with their dietary practices**.[34,35]

—Vanadium

In addition to chromium and magnesium, the little-known trace mineral **vanadium** also plays important roles in supporting healthy blood sugar levels as a part of the diet. In humans, dietary supplementation with vanadium supports glucose metabolism in muscle cells – promoting normally healthy blood glucose regulation.

Vitamins, Minerals and the Immune System

—Vitamin D

The many roles for **vitamin D** that have been discovered in the last decade include contributions to the strength and robustness of the immune system. For example, vitamin D has been shown in research published recently in the *Journal of Clinical Investigation* to enhance the immune system's production of small protein molecules that support the body's defenses against external immune insults.[36] Vitamin D appears to interact in a coordinated manner with cells near a new wound, strengthening the ability of the body to protect its integrity while a wound heals.

—Vitamin C

One of the major functions of vitamin C is to work with the cells of the immune system to enhance their ability to maintain our immune defenses. The day-to-day importance of this function was endorsed by the Cochrane Collaboration (an independent therapeutic assessment service whose conclusions are relied upon by many health professionals, including the American Academy of Family Physicians).[37] **After a thorough statistical re-analysis of the scientific literature, this group concluded that vitamin C supports the human immune system.**

—Zinc

The intriguing role of **zinc** as an essential trace element for immune function is well established. Zinc facilitates crosstalk and coordination of effort between the various cells of the immune system and is absolutely required in order for immune cells to rapidly replicate and multiply during an immune response. If zinc is not available in sufficient amounts, immune cell functions are compromised; for example, zinc ensures the accuracy of cellular immune marker recognition by some types of lymphocytes. In addition, the effective response of the white blood cells known as "natural killer cells" is dependent on zinc supplies. Clearly, maintaining strong zinc status promotes healthy immune system functioning. Because the ability of the human immune system to adapt to new challenges has been shown to decline with increasing age, the importance of healthy zinc nutrition to healthy immune system function can have a tremendous beneficial impact on healthy aging.[38]

B-Vitamins and Energy Levels

—Thiamin, Riboflavin, Niacin, Pantothenic Acid, Biotin

Most of the B-vitamins are required for the conversion of sugars and fats into energy that can be used by the body. Thiamin, riboflavin, niacin, pantothenic acid and biotin are all indispensable for these processes and the rate at which the body can produce usable energy will be set by the B-vitamin that is the least abundant.[40]

Inadequate intakes of the B-vitamins results in classical symptoms of energy deficiency, with the tissues that are affected reflecting those that are the most sensitive to any particular individual B-vitamin.[40] Stark signs and symptoms of B-vitamin deficiencies are well-known. Without getting into the nitty-gritty, thiamin deficiency can influence nerve, brain and heart function, riboflavin deficiency has consequences for the skin and nerves, niacin deficiency can impact mental health, the skin and bowel health, pantothenic acid deficiency also impacts the skin, liver and can influence blood sugar regulation, while biotin is needed for healthy connective tissue such as skin, hair and nails.

—Folate, Vitamin B_{12}

Two B-vitamins play special roles in support of the production of red blood cells.[40] Poor intakes of folate or vitamin B_{12} will cause new red blood cell production to slow. As old red blood cells are removed from the circulation, a reduction in the rate of replacement will impair the blood's ability to deliver oxygen to cells, and loss of endurance will result.

Vitamins, Minerals and Dental Health

—Vitamin C

The need for **vitamin C** to allow the tough fibers of the gums to link together is the most famous example of the way an essential component of the diet is irreplaceable in the maintenance of human health. The recognition of this role founded the science of vitaminology. By promoting strong and healthy gums, vitamin C contributes to dental health.

—Magnesium, Calcium and Vitamin D

Strong teeth require more than just strong gums – they also need strong underlying bone through which they attach to the gums and the jawbone. Of course, sound **calcium** and **vitamin D** nutrition will allow those stalwarts of bone health to foster dental longevity. In addition, it is becoming clear that there is another, underappreciated member of the dental health team – **magnesium**. As shown in one survey of adults, **the greater the daily intake of magnesium, the better the health of the periodontal tissue.**[41]

Vitamins, Minerals and Healthy Aging Go Hand-In-Hand

It's obvious that the old way of seeing vitamins – as simple helpers – can no longer stand the light of day. Each vitamin plays multiple roles in contributing to human health. Minerals also deserve their own places in the promotion of healthy aging. Look to an advanced multivitamin and multimineral formulation that combines state-of-the-art manufacturing, is based on the latest science, delivers balanced and adequate amounts, especially of the nutrients you're most likely to need more of – magnesium and vitamin D. Think of your multivitamin and multimineral formula as the foundation of your Healthy Aging program. Choosing a high-quality formulation will pay dividends for years to come.

While stark and absolute deficiencies of any of these essential nutrients results in overt problems with health, even minor deficiencies can have health consequences. Beyond that, these nutrients have health benefits in excess as well, as they support the integrity of the antioxidant system and can substitute for other nutrients when demand is high. Vitamins and minerals are not just the most essential of the nutrients, but also the most versatile of nature's tools designed to help you age enjoyably, gracefully and in the very best of health.

Section II

Healthy Aging -
A Systems-Based Approach
to Achieving Optimal
Health

11

Dietary Choices: Establishing a Foundation for Health

It is abundantly clear that our dietary habits are the most intimate predictors of our long-term health. From the foods we consume, our body extracts vitamins and minerals, fats, carbohydrates and proteins, and other necessary components that support all aspects of its metabolism. This process is only as good as the input provided. If we eat healthfully, and the foods we eat are nutrient-dense, the body is able to extract a majority of what it needs for health directly from our diet. In contrast, if the majority of what we eat is unhealthy, and the food we eat is empty calories with little or no nutritional value, there is a great propensity to develop deficiencies of key nutrients that impact the body's metabolic functions. Thus, the key is not how much we eat; it most certainly is the type of foods we consume.

The Basics

The fundamentals of a good diet begin with eating food that provides the body what it needs to function optimally. First and foremost, this includes making dietary choices that give the most bang for your buck, nutritionally speaking. As the essential components of the diet are proteins, carbohydrates and fats, making wise choices by selecting the most healthful types of these nutritional building blocks can go a long way in promoting health.

Protein is a major building block for the body in that it is necessary for immune function, growth and development. Our muscle mass is composed of protein, and antibodies, enzymes and hormones are protein-based. Adequate protein intake also serves to stabilize blood sugar levels. Thus, it is essential to ensure optimal intake of protein as well as to eat sources of protein that contain a full complement of amino acids. Good sources of protein include meats, fish, poultry, dairy products and eggs as well as various vegetarian sources of protein including beans, nuts, seeds, and legumes. Eating a variety of healthy protein-containing foods ensures the body has the amino acid building blocks that are necessary for cell and tissue repair.

Carbohydrates are important for energy production. They can be divided into two major groups - simple carbohydrates and complex carbohydrates. Simple carbohydrates consist of the simple sugars such as sucrose, fructose, lactose and others, and are also found in fruits. Complex carbohydrates are found in foods such as vegetables, beans, nuts, seeds and whole grains. Simple carbohydrates are broken down and metabolized faster than complex carbohydrates, which consist of longer chains. Simple carbohydrates raise blood glucose levels more quickly than complex carbohydrates. Depending on an individual's activity levels, a diet consisting of more simple or more complex carbohydrates can be necessary. However, intake of more complex carbohydrates is usually more beneficial since it raises blood sugar levels more slowly, avoiding spikes and crashes due to varying blood sugar levels. Complex carbohydrate-rich foods also tend to be healthier as simple carbohydrates are present in large amounts in most processed foods. Dietary fiber contained in fruits and vegetables is also a complex carbohydrate that isn't metabolized or digested by the body but contributes to health in many important ways. Unrefined, unprocessed foods are often highest in dietary fiber and are therefore healthier choices.

Fat is also an essential component of a healthy diet. Fat provides a concentrated form of energy for the body and is necessary for normal brain development. However, excessive fat intake has been linked to obesity and several diseases. It turns out that the type of fat consumed determines its likely effects on health. Fats consist of saturated fats, primarily found in animal products, and polyunsaturated and monounsaturated fats, generally found in most plant foods. Fish is an excellent source of polyunsaturated fatty acids as well. While excessive intake of saturated fats can raise blood cholesterol levels, the "healthy" polyunsaturated and monounsaturated fats may lower blood levels of cholesterol. Another adverse contributor to unhealthy cholesterol levels are the *trans*-fatty acids. These occur as a consequence of the process of hydrogenation of vegetable oils, such as in the production of margarine. These fats can raise cholesterol levels, particularly levels of bad cholesterol, while reducing levels of good protective HDL cholesterol levels. Needless to say, they should be avoided.

Environmental Factors and Food Additives

Along with the notion that high quality and healthier types of proteins, carbohydrates and fats should be eaten preferentially, consideration should also be given to eating "clean" foods such as those that are organic and those devoid of synthetic pesticides, chemicals and hormones. Eating these foods is healthier for the body as they tend to be higher in nutritional value and easier for the body to process, as it has to devote fewer resources to detoxifying the synthetic chemicals and unnatural compounds that can themselves have detrimental effects on the body's physiology. Choosing organic fruits and vegetables when possible, as well as free-range meats and wild-caught seafood, can ultimately improve health.

Just as important as any of the macronutrients discussed, is the necessity of consuming water. As our bodies are two-thirds water, decreased water consumption (which can lead to dehydration) can adversely affect the numerous metabolic processes the body undergoes on a daily basis. Water is essential to the body's detoxification systems and is a critical component of all cells. Furthermore, water is involved in digestion, circulation, absorption of nutrients and the maintenance of proper electrolyte balance. The consumption of adequate amounts of pure water ensures the health of all cells and tissues.

> *"Choosing organic fruits and vegetables when possible, as well as free-range meats and wild-caught seafood, can ultimately improve health."*

When it comes to a healthy diet, the bottom line is to ensure we eat nutrient-dense foods that contain healthy proteins, carbohydrates and fats, providing essential vitamins and minerals, consume whole foods that are free of synthetic pesticides, chemicals and hormones, and take in adequate amounts of pure, fresh water. By avoiding processed foods and beverages, we can eliminate excessive consumption of simple carbohydrates and sugars and foods with additives and artificial ingredients. Sticking to a diet composed mainly of whole natural foods leads to healthier outcomes in the long run.

There are many models of traditionally healthy dietary habits that have been employed by cultures throughout the world. One such dietary concept is the Mediterranean model. In fact, recently there has been a tremendous amount of interest in the so-called "Mediterranean Diet" and its value in health promotion. This dietary lifestyle first caught the attention of nutritionists because it seems to violate a fundamental dogma of modern nutrition – it has a high total fat content!

Yet study after study has shown less heart disease and fewer cancers among population groups that practice this dietary lifestyle.[1,2] So what is it about this "diet" high in total fat that leads it to be so seemingly healthy?

The Mediterranean Diet

The term, "Mediterranean Diet," implying that all Mediterranean people have the same diet, is a misnomer. The peoples of the Mediterranean region have a variety of diets, religions and cultures, and their diets differ somewhat in fat, olive oil, meat, wine, fruit, vegetable and dairy product contents. What most people think of when they hear the phrase, "Mediterranean Diet," actually is the traditional diet of Greece prior to 1960.[3] Nonetheless, the concept of a "Mediterranean Diet" has become a permanent part of the public consciousness.

> *"Dietary lifestyle patterns that now are considered to be reflective of the Mediterranean Diet include the consumption of abundant amounts of fruits, vegetables, fish, whole grain breads, beans, nuts and seeds."*

Dietary lifestyle patterns that now are considered to be reflective of the Mediterranean Diet include the consumption of abundant amounts of fruits, vegetables, fish, whole grain breads, beans, nuts and seeds.[1,3] The fruits and vegetables usually are fresh, minimally processed, and grown relatively locally (with little commercial shipping). Concentrated simple sugars and processed flour products are avoided. In contrast to westernized practices, the major source of dietary fats is olive oil. Eggs, cheese, yogurt and lean red meats are consumed only occasionally and milk is avoided. Wine (more often, red wine) is consumed with restraint and with meals. These principles mirror many of those we discussed early on in this section regarding tips for generally healthy dietary practices.

The Mediterranean Diet and Health Benefits – What Does the Data Say?

The results of a large number of studies all point in the same direction – the eating practices of individuals on the "Mediterranean Diet" keep people healthier.

The results of an analysis that combined the findings of many studies in an attempt to find the patterns that have emerged was published recently in *Nutrition Reviews*.[1] The paper considered all of the possible health benefits that could be obtained from this lifestyle. These researchers concluded that the "Mediterranean Diet" does indeed keep people healthier. People who lived this lifestyle their entire lives as well as people who adopted it during participation in a research study enjoyed lower serum total and low-density lipoprotein-cholesterol (LDL-cholesterol) concentrations, lower plasma triglycerides, higher serum high-density-cholesterol (HDL-cholesterol) concentrations, greater total plasma antioxidant capacity, more responsive and compliant blood vessels, greater insulin sensitivity and tighter blood glucose control, less cardiovascular disease, fewer heart attacks, fewer and milder joint problems, a tendency to lower body fatness and fewer cancers.

These conclusions repeat those that were reached previously by other experts.[4] Those earlier scientists concluded that a shift to the traditional healthy Mediterranean diet by people living in highly developed Western countries could reduce by 10% to 25% the occurrence of cancers of the colon, rectum, breast, prostate, pancreas and endometrium.

Another investigator has published the results of a more detailed examination of the specifics of the Mediterranean dietary lifestyle in the scientific journal, *Public Health Nutrition*, in an article titled, "Mediterranean Diet and Cancer."[5] This public health expert concluded that individuals who regularly consume at least 5 servings of fruits, at least 5 servings of vegetables, at least 1 serving of fish, at least one serving of whole grains and at least two tablespoons of olive oil (high in monounsaturated fats) every day, while eating red meat no more often than once every other day, would cut in half their chances of ever developing cancer of the mouth, throat, esophagus, stomach, colon, rectum, liver, gallbladder, pancreas, kidney, urinary bladder or prostate (if male) or breast, endometrium or ovary (if female).

The results of a recently-completed "gold standard" randomized controlled clinical trial, published in the *Annals of Internal Medicine,* are consistent with all of the previous conclusions and predictions concerning the health benefits of this lifestyle. In this study, two versions of the Mediterranean dietary lifestyle, differing in major fat source, were compared to a standard low-fat diet.[6] Regardless of whether the additional dietary fat was in the form of olive oil or nuts, both versions of the Mediterranean dietary lifestyle produced much tighter control of blood glucose concentrations, promoted normalization of blood pressure, lowered serum LDL-cholesterol concentrations and reduced signs of systemic inflammation.

Beneficial effects on body weight probably contribute to these positive outcomes. As shown in the results of a study of over 3,000 men and women living in northeastern Spain, the closer an individual adheres to this lifestyle, the less likely he or she is to become overweight.[7]

Is It The Oil?

A mainstay of the Mediterranean dietary lifestyle is the copious use and consumption of high-quality extra virgin cold-pressed olive oil. Is this important? The results of a recently-published randomized controlled clinical trial has shown that the high phytonutrient content of extra virgin olive oil is "heart healthy," producing increased serum HDL-cholesterol concentrations and decreased serum triglyceride, LDL-cholesterol and oxidized LDL-cholesterol concentrations.[8] In addition, a laboratory study has shown that two of the polyphenol phytonutrients in olive oil, hydroxytyrosol and oleuropein, impair the ability of damaged blood vessel lining cells to trick white blood cells into helping them form an arterial plaque.[9]

These findings help explain the observation that the routine, life-long consumption of several tablespoons of high-quality olive oil daily (as salad dressing, cooking oil, salsa or olives) can reduce the chances of ever having a heart attack by 75% or more.[10]

Of course, the health benefits of olive oil extend far beyond the heart and cardiovascular system. For example a recently published review article demonstrated that breast cancer and colon cancer in particular are less likely to occur in adults who habitually practice a Mediterranean dietary lifestyle.[2] These reviewers explained the mechanisms through which oleic acid, the major monounsaturated fatty acid (MUFA) in olive oil, suppressed several of the very first biochemical events that convert a normal breast or colon cell into a cancerous cell – a mechanism that could help oncologists understand better the value of olive oil both to their patients and as a "cancer preventive" option for the general population.

> "Of course, the health benefits of olive oil extend far beyond the heart and cardiovascular system."

Is It The Wine?

Another vital component of the Mediterranean dietary lifestyle is the enjoyment of one or two glasses of wine in moderation, usually red, every day (or nearly so). Can red wine be another link between the Mediterranean dietary lifestyle and good health?

Many scientists have examined this question during the last decade. They have found that the regular daily consumption of one or two glasses of red wine, once a day during or just after a meal, can:

- reduce the risk of having a heart attack by about 50%.
- reduce the likelihood of developing congestive heart failure by about 50%
- cut the chances of dying from heart disease or cancer by up to 50%.

More recently, a group of European investigators have published in the scientific journal, *Physiological Research*, the results of a formal analysis of the tremendous volume of scientific research linking red wine to cardiovascular health.[11] They concluded that red wine:

- reduces the ability of arterial plaques to form or enlarge
- reduces the ability of arterial plaques to cause narrowing of the arteries
- increases the health of heart muscle
- increases resistance to developing high blood pressure

These conclusions are consistent with the results obtained by this group in their own research, as published in the journal *Physiological Research*.[12]

Finally, a group of Canadian cardiologists have "said it all" in their summary assessment published recently in the *American Journal of Physiology*.[13] These experts have concluded that the consumption of one or two glasses of red wine, once a day during or just after a meal, can markedly reduce your chances of ever suffering from:

- heart attack
- angina
- congestive heart failure
- stroke
- coronary artery blockages
- atherosclerotic plaques
- vascular thrombosis
- peripheral arterial disease
- intermittent claudication
- hypertension

How can Red Wine be so beneficial?

Scientists know that when you drink a glass of red wine, for the next day or so you have decreased:

- susceptibility of the cholesterol-laden lipoprotein particles in your blood to become oxidized.
- susceptibility of the monocyte cells in your blood to become converted into plaque-forming cells.
- release of monocyte-attracting chemicals by the cells lining the inner walls of your blood vessels.
- migration of blood monocytes to the linings of the inner walls of your blood vessels.
- ability of blood monocytes to attach to the linings of the inner walls of your blood vessels.
- conversion of blood monocytes into cholesterol-laden foam cells within the inner walls of your blood vessels.

and increased:

- resistance to stimuli that cause uncontrolled proliferation of the cells that line your blood vessels (which results in less narrowing of those vessels).
- resistance to stimuli that cause uncontrolled proliferation of the smooth muscle cells that wrap around your blood vessels and control their diameter (which results in less narrowing and stiffness of blood vessels – major causes of high blood pressure).

The Mediterranean Diet Will Benefit Your Health

What does this mean for us? The jury's still out. However, one thing seems clear - the "Mediterranean Diet", can certainly enhance health and well-being and may be protective of the heart, arteries, brains, muscles and numerous other tissues. The Mediterranean dietary lifestyle is health-promoting and life-enhancing.

The Mediterranean Diet – Can you do it?

There is no reason why we all can't incorporate more of the health-promoting dietary practices as advocated by the "Mediterranean Diet" into our daily lives. This requires increased emphasis on fresh foods and may require increased efforts in food preparation, which is not that appealing or convenient. When eating out, it requires thinking about making healthier choices.

All of these apparent obstacles can be overcome if you are serious about your health and simply make up your mind to live a healthier lifestyle. Once you decide to improve your health by adopting healthful dietary practices, you need to make a plan. Start by taking small steps towards eating better by making gradual changes that are in line with the recommendations provided here. Don't bite off more than you can chew. That may lead to frustration if you're not able to follow through completely. Making incremental changes over a period of time leads to better compliance. If you fall off the wagon occasionally, don't beat yourself up over it. Just get back on and move forward. Healthy eating leads to healthy bodies.

> *"...one thing seems clear - consumption of foods rich in resveratrol and other phytonutrients, as in the "Mediterranean Diet", can certainly enhance health and well-being and may be protective of the heart, arteries, brains, muscles and numerous other tissues."*

12

Exercise, Health and Longevity

The research is clear: Regular exercise extends human life. Among the data confirming this observation are the results of the Harvard Alumni Health Study.[1] Over the 15 years during which these 13,486 men were studied, age at death was increased significantly in proportion to the distance walked daily, the number of stories of stairs climbed daily and the amount of vigorous physical exercise that was included in each day's activities. Another study of 19,223 initially healthy men found that cardiorespiratory fitness reduced both the incidence of premature death and the incidence of death from cardiovascular disease by 54%.[2]

> "Regular exercise extends human life."

The close relationship between physical activity and life extension was confirmed by the 24-year prospective Nurses' Health Study.[3] Among these 116,564 women in the US, increasing the amount of routine physical activity performed daily decreased the chances of dying prematurely, with the decrease first appearing when regular physical activity exceeds 3.5 hours per week. These investigators estimated that the combination of smoking cessation, maintaining BMI below 26 and participation in regular physical activity in excess of 3.5 hours per week could prevent 31% of all premature deaths.

One group of investigators concluded that increasing the amount of routine physical activity can reduce the risk for premature death by about one quarter.[4] Another group estimated that "at least 30 minutes of moderate physical activity on most days of the week" can reduce the risk of premature death by about one-third.[5]

Among a 69,693-woman subset of the Nurses' Health Study, the likelihood of suffering a heart attack was doubled in women who habitually failed to exercise at least twice weekly, while 4 or more hours of exercise a week cut the risk of dying from a heart attack in half.[6] The cardioprotective properties of regular habitual exercise also are apparent in men; in the 12-year prospective Physicians' Health Study, the chances of dying from a heart attack were reduced by 85% in men who habitually exercised at least 5 times weekly.[7] The data collected during that study indicate that simply running for one hour per week or lifting weights for 30 minutes once a week reduces the chances of developing heart disease.[8] Similarly in the US, the Women's Health Initiative Observational Study of 73,743 postmenopausal women observed a 20% decrease in the incidence of cardiovascular disease among women who exercised routinely.[9] Other scientists have concluded that, on average, the likelihood of dying from heart disease is about 90% greater in sedentary adults than in those who are physically active.[10]

The author of a comprehensive examination of the health benefits of physical activity, published recently in *Australian Family Physician* concluded that a 40-minute session of resistance exercise, only once or twice a week (but at least 48 hours apart to allow for maximum muscle recovery and growth) will increase strength and neuromuscular coordination in older men and women.[11] Greater strength and coordination will improve mobility and will make stumbling and falling – and breaking bones – less likely. The risk of fractures is exceedingly high with advancing age. Weight-bearing exercise is critical for retaining healthy bone density and strengthening bone matrix. Healthier bones lead to a decreased risk of osteoporotic bone fractures.

Regular Exercise Reduces Systemic Inflammation

Exercise also contributes to the health of the entire body – even those "parts" not involved in the exercise itself. Scientific evidence presented in an article published recently in the *Journal of Applied Physiology* demonstrates that because exercise increases the secretion of the anti-inflammatory cytokine, interleukin-6 (IL-6), by muscle cells into the blood stream, and IL-6 inhibits the secretion of the pro-inflammatory cytokine, tumor necrosis factor- (TNF-) throughout the body, regular participation in physical activity will decrease the level of disease-causing inflammation throughout the body.[12]

Regular Exercise Reduces Cancer Risk

Several specific examples of the positive benefits of regular exercise on inflammation and the immune system are obvious. The scientific evidence is consistent: the enormous amount of data collected from the 51,529 men who participated in the Health Professionals Follow-Up Study and the 121,701 women who participated in the Nurses' Health Study confirm that regular participation in physical activity cuts the chances of developing cancer of the colon or pancreas by half.[13-15] In its 2006 "white paper," published in the *Journal of Clinical Oncology*, the American Society of Clinical Oncology concluded that regular exercise decreases the chances that a women will develop breast cancer and decreases the chances that a breast cancer survivor will suffer a recurrence.[16]

According to the results of a recently published study, participation in regular physical activity has been proven to slow down the rate at which existing prostate cancer worsens.[17] Women benefit, too – research published recently in the *Journal of the American Medical Association* found that one hour of regular physical activity daily increases the survival of women with breast cancer.[18] Further research demonstrates that one hour of regular physical activity daily increases the quality of life and decreases fatigue in breast cancer survivors.[19]

Regular Exercise Reduces ALL Disease Risk

The author of a comprehensive examination of the health benefits of physical activity concluded that "there is irrefutable evidence of the effectiveness of regular physical activity in the primary and secondary prevention of cardiovascular disease, diabetes, cancer, hypertension, obesity, depression, osteoporosis and premature death."[20] The greater the increase in physical fitness, the greater the reduction in the risk of premature death. Overall, doubling the exercise capacity of an individual reduces the risk of premature death by about 50%.

> *"Doubling the exercise capacity of an individual reduces the risk of premature death by about 50%."*

Regular Exercise Enhances the Quality of Old Age

One of the greatest fears of adults is reaching old age in a debilitated, dysfunctional condition – riddled with disease and on multiple medications. Aging this way is not necessary — by slowing down the march to diseases and debilitating conditions, doubling your musculoskeletal fitness can delay the onset of loss of functional independence by 10 to 30 years.[20] Exercise significantly enhances quality of life and overall productivity.

Regular Exercise as a Key to Weight Management

Exercising on a consistent basis (along with healthy dietary practices) enhances our ability to maintain a healthy body weight. Being overweight or obese is a major factor in developing several chronic diseases. Maintaining a healthy body weight reduces our risk of developing those same diseases by reducing overall inflammation in the body.

By being overweight, we put ourselves at increased risk of diseases and conditions such as diabetes, high blood pressure, high cholesterol, heart disease, respiratory disease, sleep issues, asthma, digestive disorders, liver problems, joint conditions and arthritis, and several types of cancer.[21] Cancers of the stomach, colon, rectum, liver, gallbladder, pancreas, prostate, kidneys, breast and reproductive organs are all more common in individuals who are overweight.[22]

Establishing a regimen of regular, routine exercise can help us ensure that we burn off the excess calories we get from our diets. By helping us reach a body weight that is healthy, exercise wards off diseases and lays the foundation for health. By exercising regularly, we can all more fully experience the wonders of life in a healthier and more active state for much, much longer.

Top Tips for Longevity Enhancement through Exercise

- Get Some! It doesn't matter so much whether you walk, run, lift weights or whatever – just get moving!
- Stretch before starting and after finishing – reward your muscles for their hard work.
- Start slowly and build up speed and intensity only gradually – your engines need to warm up for best performance.
- Between 30 and 60 minutes a day, 5 or 6 days a week, is ideal for movement activities.
- If you are uncertain about how to do something, ask a pro – only if done correctly can activities benefit you.
- If you experience unusual pain, stop! Pain is nature's way of telling you something may be wrong. Check in with a medical professional.
- If something is hurting, don't push it. It will heal but you must give it time to do so. Don't be afraid to take off a few days with alternative activities. (Twist an ankle? Do arm lifts while you sit with good posture.)

- To help your muscles work better, recover more quickly and grow bigger and stronger, feed them high-quality protein and plenty of antioxidants.
- To keep your muscles well-fed, ensure you are maintaining healthy circulation.
- Make sure to get enough sleep. Sleep helps the body recover by providing it critically important down time.
- If you're not exercising now, check with your physician first about how to start.

13

Healthy Digestion: The Key to a Healthy You

The proper digestion of the foods you eat and the beverages you drink requires the integrated cooperation of vastly complex chemical and physical machinery. Only when every component is operating efficiently can your food be converted into your good health. It's amazing how integral proper digestive function is to health overall. Optimizing digestive function impacts the health of so many other systems throughout the body. We all know the saying, "You are what you eat!" This is indeed true as digestive health is the key to overall wellness.

As one thinks about this link, it makes sense. After all, the digestive tract, stretching from the mouth to the rectum, is a major site of contact with the outside world. Our food, toxins, microbes and other environmental substances all enter our system through the digestive tract. This system plays a critical role as an immune barrier in two major ways. Firstly, it acts as a structural barrier simply by keeping bad things out and good things in, only allowing things to pass through for particular reasons. Second, it's a major component of our immune system and the first line of defense for our bodies. Major immune structures and immunoglobulins reside in the digestive tract or are manufactured there. These factors play an important role in maintaining our overall immune defenses. Thus the dual role played by the digestive tract, by acting as a physical barrier and an immunological barrier, is critical to our health. Given this crucial function, it's easy to see how the health of the digestive tract can impact so many other areas throughout the body.

Now that we understand the importance of digestive health, let's look at how we can best maintain it. In order to do that, we need to explore the function of the various components of this system. Digestion literally begins with the sight and smell of food. These senses initiate the production of enzymes in the mouth that prepare for the arrival of food and to begin the process of breaking foods down. Of course, chewing is a critically important step as this allows the salivary enzymes to begin acting on the food. From here, the food moves down through the esophagus and into the stomach.

> *"Our food, toxins, microbes and other environmental substances all enter our system through the digestive tract."*

Stomach

The stomach mixes food with the acid and enzymes it adds to what you've eaten; the acid partially dissolves big food particles into much smaller ones and the enzymes begin the digestion of those smaller fat and protein particles. Along with stomach acid, pepsin plays an important role by breaking down proteins into smaller particles known as peptides.

Small Intestine

The small intestine is where most food digestion and nutrient absorption occur. Most food digestion occurs in the upper small intestine and most of the absorption of the individual nutrients occurs in its lower regions. Anything remaining after traveling down the length of the small intestine goes into the large intestine for a different kind of processing before being expelled in the stool.

Pancreatic Enzymes

Food leaving the stomach stimulates the pancreas to send a package of digestive enzymes to the small intestine where they join the bile from the gallbladder. Together these enzymes can digest just about anything we're likely to eat except fiber. They serve to further break down fats, carbohydrates and proteins into their components and nutrients for assimilation. But there's a catch – all of the digesting compounds sent to the small intestine could digest our pancreas and gall bladder, so they are initially sent in inactive forms. Once they arrive, the small intestine releases a "master enzyme" that activates all of the others and gets digestion really rolling.

Bicarbonate

There's another catch – all that stomach acid could deactivate the enzymes. To prevent this, the pancreas sends along with its enzymes some bicarbonate. This neutralizes the excess acidity and serves to protect the enzymes and lining of the small intestine from stomach acids. The small intestine itself does its part by covering its inner lining with a layer of bicarbonate-rich mucus.

Water

In order for the digestive process to function smoothly, water is a necessary cofactor. Copious amounts of water are needed to keep everything dissolved. This water comes from the beverages we drink during meals and snacks and from your blood. Several cups of water are moved from your circulation into your digestive tract with each meal or snack. While in younger people the hydration of the circulation is maintained by the entry of water from other parts of the body, studies published recently in the *American Journal of Clinical Nutrition* and the *Journal of Applied* found that in older adults the body surrenders less of its total water to the circulation, increasing the risk for bouts of dehydration after meals.[1,2]

The Colon

Your large intestine, or colon, is required to perform one major and essential task above all others – retrieve back into the body the water that has been added to your food by your saliva and digestive secretions. This water was taken from your bloodstream (about 1 to 2 cups per meal) and added to the material in your alimentary tract (the "digesta") to help your body digest food and absorb its nutrients relatively rapidly and, for the most part, extremely efficiently. However, if that water is simply lost through your stool you would dehydrate very rapidly a few hours after every meal – certainly not a healthy outcome!

The cells lining the colon are responsible for recapturing the water and restoring it to your blood. Normally they are very efficient. And, like anybody else, these hard workers need to be fed. Here's something you probably don't know: Unlike just about every other cell in our body, the cells lining our colon are not fed through the bloodstream. They get their nutrition directly from whatever gets to them from the small intestine - the leftovers of the digestive process. If they are undernourished, they cannot operate effectively. This leads to abnormal stools and inefficient digestive function.

> *"Maintaining healthy gut ecology by supporting colon health is necessary for our well-being."*

Recently, the colon has also been recognized as a major immune organ. It contributes to overall immunity by functioning as the reservoir for healthy (and unfortunately, unhealthy) bacteria and yeast. Numerous studies shine light on the positive health benefits associated with healthy gut ecology and adequate numbers and strains of probiotic organisms. Likewise, the chronic presence of unhealthy bacteria and yeast lead to unhealthy digestive function and detrimental effects on immune functioning. Maintaining healthy gut ecology by supporting colon health is necessary for our well-being.

Our colon depends on two major factors to keep it healthy: 1) A healthy balance of probiotic organisms, as the intestines, particularly the colon, are where the majority of these beneficial organisms reside, and 2) Sufficient amounts of fiber in the diet. This should be in the form of both soluble and insoluble fibers.

Changes with Age

Research suggests that this entire process may work less and less well as we get older. And of course there's no justice – this age effect doesn't mean we can eat more without gaining as much weight; it means that as we age the balance between what we eat, what we absorb and what our body needs grows increasingly out of whack. Thus, with age it becomes more necessary to ensure that our digestive tracts function at an optimal level. This often requires nutritional support.

Optimize Your Digestion

Stomach Acid

Make sure that your stomach is doing its job to prepare food for further digestion. Stomach acid production may decrease with age. There are tests your doctor can do to measure how well your stomach produces acid during digestion. However, one way to estimate this is by looking at the nature of your stool. If you regularly see some undigested food (other than certain nuts, seeds and corn, which can be normal) – that's right, it's OK to look – you might want to consider adding a small acid tablet (in the form of **Betaine HCl**) to the middle of large meals. Often times, Betaine HCl will be combined with the enzyme pepsin and may also include bitter herbs such as Gentian, which can stimulate the digestive process. Choose a high quality product or, if you are unsure, check with a nutritionally oriented physician.

Digestive Enzymes

Like stomach acid, age and other factors can affect our body's ability to produce sufficient digestive enzymes. If these aren't available in large enough amounts, some of our food will not be digested and you may not enjoy the complete benefits of healthy nutrition from your diet. Research published recently in the *Scandinavian Journal of Gastroenterology* found that between 5% and 10% of all adults in their 50's suffered some decrease in the amount of digestive enzymes they produced and that over 15% suffered some decrease by their 70's.[3] In order to counteract this, individuals can add spices to their food. In fact, spices provide health benefits far beyond their digestive properties.

Many spices, including cinnamon, curcumin, coriander, fennel, garlic, ginger and tamarind (major components of foods such as curry), are known to stimulate the production of bile acids and digestive enzymes. If some undigested food still appears regularly in your stool – that's right, you need to look again – you also might want to consume (with some water) a dietary supplement containing a mixture of digestive enzymes either before or during meals.

Keep Your Inner Insides Wet

Drinking fluids as you eat helps reduce the amount of "drying" that must occur in your bloodstream. However, be cautious with this. In the Ayurvedic and Unani systems of traditional medicine, drinking large amounts of water or liquids with meals is thought to reduce "digestive capacity". Again, in traditional medical systems, this method of drinking fluids slowly over a period of time is thought to encourage absorption of the fluid by cells and tissues whereas drinking fluid in large amounts may simply lead to excessive urination. In addition, drinking plenty of fluids between meals and snacks allows your body to remain fully hydrated and maintain a reserve of extra water that can be available for perspiration and participation in the digestive process.[4]

Loosen Up

Not too surprisingly, research has demonstrated that tight-fitting clothing, especially compressive undergarments, interferes with nutrient digestion and can prevent you from enjoying all of the benefits of a good diet.[5]

Intestinal Antioxidants and Fuel

The small protein **glutathione** is the major antioxidant protecting your intestinal cells from the oxidative damage that can be inflicted by the byproducts of the massive amount of digestive chemistry going on all around them. Some portion of an oral supplement of glutathione is broken down by digestive enzymes before it can be absorbed, between 2% and 10% is absorbed, and the remainder acts along the lining of the gut to protect gut cells from the "collateral damage" that can be caused by the digestive processes. Since it seems that so little of oral glutathione is actually absorbed, supplementing with nutrients that increase the body's own production of glutathione may be more beneficial. One such nutrient is the amino acid glutamine. Glutamine is a key component of the glutathione molecule and, as shown in a study published very recently in the *Journal of Nutritional Biochemistry*, supplemental glutamine can stimulate the self-protective synthesis of glutathione by gut cells.[6] Even more amazingly, intestinal cells rely on glutamine, not glucose or fatty acids, for most of their energy needs. Combined supplementation with nutrients that enhance glutathione production such as glutamine can help promote a healthy intestinal tract by defusing the oxidizing byproducts of digestion.

Probiotics, Prebiotics and Fiber

Adequate amounts of dietary fiber are essential to overall digestive health and colonic function. Likewise, probiotics are also essential to overall digestive wellness, colon health and a healthy immune system. An unhealthy colon leads to many things. One of the first manifestations is abnormal bowel movements.

Consistency of Bowel Movements

As one of the most fundamental functions of the colon is maintaining water balance, it performs this function by affecting the consistency of the stool. When colon cells are starving they are not able to shift water from the lumen of the colon back to the blood. The water stays in the gut and leaves (usually somewhat hurriedly) as a wet or even really watery stool – that's **diarrhea**. Once that happens, you're dehydrated, and your upper digestive tract adds less water to the materials it is trying to digest. Because they contain less water, these materials do not "slide" along the gut as easily and they tend to clog the digestive tube. By the time they reach the colon, they may have formed a mass that is too hard to deform by colon muscle contractions – this mass then tends to stay put – that's **constipation**. This vicious cycle illustrates two extremes of an unhealthy colon.

One of two things then happens: either you manage somehow to pass this dry hard stool or you take a laxative that contains a chemical that forces your colon to contract so hard that it expels the lump. In both situations, the cells lining the colon and rectum can become irritated. Now, because less water was "wasted" in this bowel movement, your body has a chance to re-establish water balance. But your colon is now irritated in addition to being underfed. The next time your colon receives material from the small intestine, it "takes back" even less of the water, leading to another episode of dehydrating diarrhea. And so on. In many adults who do not realize that this is both abnormal and correctable through the diet, this cycle can perpetuate for years and even decades. In order to break this cycle, we need to ensure that the colon is being "fed" with the nutrients it needs.

> "...probiotics are also essential to overall digestive wellness, colon health and a healthy immune system."

In order to remain healthy, the colon cells thrive by eating the leftovers from our diet. In short – whatever remains after the bacteria, yeast, molds and protozoa in the colon have had their fill. Remember, not much ingested material reaches the colon – only about 10% or less of an average meal. As a function of normal digestion, by the time these leftovers get to your colon, almost all of the nutrients have been removed by the small intestine.

It is reassuring to know that the microbial residents of your colon are much better at chemically converting the material that reaches the colon into useful nutrients than they are at gobbling up those nutrients, so there can be plenty left-over for your colon cells to enjoy. Thus healthy bacteria do their part in maintaining the symbiotic relationship with our bodies, benefiting them and us. In addition to the vitamins and amino acids produced and shared by the microbes, the most important product of their activity for the health of colon cells is the conversion of undigested foodstuffs into what are called **short-chain fatty acids**.

Short-Chain Fatty Acids – Gourmet Food for the Colon

The most important of the short-chain fatty acids produced by colonic bacteria is butyrate.[7] The cells lining the interior surface of the human colon convert butyrate into an even smaller fatty acid (acetate) that they can burn for energy and use as a structural building material to seal the junctions between adjacent cells – strengthening the integrity of the colonic barrier and preventing the leakage of any toxins from the colon contents from entering the bloodstream. Without enough butyrate coming from the microbes within the colon, your colon cells go hungry – and the cellular junction can become compromised.

Butyrate and Cell-cycle Control

Butyrate also has another rather amazing function in human colon cells - it helps them remember that they must die, and die on time. This is vital to our ability to continue living. The concentrated exposure of our colon cells to toxins, pesticides and other contaminants entering our body makes these cells highly susceptible to oxidative damage. With enough butyrate to make acetate to seal the body off from the colon contents, your colon cells are better protected from harm.[7]

However, even in the presence of adequate butyrate, some colon cells do become damaged by free radicals. Fortunately, the biological clock ticking in every colon cell comes to the rescue – each cell is normally endowed with the ability to commit preplanned biochemical suicide (a process called "apoptosis"). Once dead, the cell remnant will detach from the colon lining and will leave with the stool, a process that ensures that colon health remains vibrant. Each cell that is lost this way is replaced by a healthy fresh new cell from the deep layers of the colon lining, and with any luck this cell will live out its life without any problems.[7] This normal process of cellular renewal ensures that the healthy integrity of colonic function is maintained.

One of the determinants of the rate of colonic cell renewal is the amount of butyrate available in the colon. Too little and the internal clock slows down, meaning the cell lives longer than it should. This is not a desirable outcome. Healthy tissues are dependent on the vitality provided by the process of cellular regeneration and renewal. A cell that is damaged by free radicals has trouble performing its normal functions and actually can facilitate a decrease in colonic health. This potentially leads to undesirable consequences. Butyrate encourages the normal, healthy lifecycle of colon cells.

Where Does the Butyrate Come From?

Butyrate is not produced by human cells. It is produced by enzymes, secreted by beneficial colonic bacteria; they chemically convert **dietary fiber** into the short chain fatty acids – most importantly, butyrate. The term "dietary fiber" actually covers a very broad category of large molecules made by plants. These molecules provide both firmness and flexibility to plants, allowing them to bend but not break in a storm. These molecules reach the colon because humans can't digest them – they pass through the mouth, throat, stomach and small intestine relatively intact.[8]

Dietary Fiber

There are several types of dietary fibers.[8] Nutritionists classify the types of dietary fibers that can be converted into butyrate as either soluble or insoluble. Examples of soluble dietary fiber include the beta-glucans (including arabinogalactans and lactoferrin), gums, mucilages, oligosaccharides and pectins. Soluble dietary fiber comprises 10% to 20% of the total dietary fiber content of such foods as fruit, okra, beans, turnips, oats, parsnips, sea weeds, and prunes. Examples of insoluble dietary fiber include the celluloses and lignins. They are found in more fibrous foods. Because it exhibits variable characteristics, a type of dietary fiber called hemicellulose is classified as both soluble and insoluble.

The soluble dietary fibers are the most readily "fermentable" in the human colon, meaning that it is easier for the normal bacterial flora to convert them into other nutrients, including butyrate. Fermentable dietary fiber serves as a "pre-biotic" in that it promotes the growth and viability of beneficial species of gut bacteria. However, dietary fiber has benefits for humans beyond the fermentability by colonic bacteria. The results of a study published recently in the *Journal of Nutrition* show that different kinds of dietary fiber can bind to glucose and fats in the digestive tract, preventing their absorption into the blood, regardless of their "solubility."[9] Fiber thus can influence the maintenance of healthy blood sugar levels and cholesterol.

Another type of dietary fiber, non-fermentable dietary fiber, is found in such foods as oat hulls, methylcellulose and wood pulp cellulose. These food components are not processed by microbes to any appreciable extent. Instead, they function in the human colon to carry the fermenting bacteria along through the colon and rectum; decrease the absorption of glucose in the small intestine and increase the glucose content of stool; dilute pathogens and toxins in the digesta and stool; distend the colonic mucosa, stimulating peristaltic contractions and increasing the rate of movement of the digesta through the digestive tract (an increased "rate of passage" decreases the amount of time that colon cells are exposed to any toxins in the digesta); and inhibit the induction of inflammation in the colon by unhealthy organisms. By promoting stool bulk, this type of fiber maintains gut ecology and supports healthy colonic function.

> *"...different kinds of dietary fiber can bind to glucose and fats in the digestive tract, preventing their absorption into the blood, regardless of their 'solubility'".*

How Much Dietary Fiber Does Your Colon Need Us to Eat?

According to the Institute of Medicine of the National Academies of Science in its dietary advisory, Dietary Reference Intakes for Energy, Carbohydrate, Fiber, Fat, Fatty Acids, Cholesterol, Protein, and Amino Acids (Macronutrients), Chapter 7: Dietary, Functional, and Total Fiber, most adults should consume 25 g to 38 g of dietary fiber daily.[10] This recommendation was based on the Institute's determination that this amount of dietary fiber could protect an individual from developing coronary artery disease. The Institute assumed that this amount also would be sufficient to promote bowel health.

Interestingly, the results of an analysis of the combined data obtained in the 76,947-woman Nurses' Health Study and the 47,279-man Health Professionals Follow-Up Study also support the concept that adequate dietary fiber intake is absolutely necessary for colon health. As a result of their analyses these scientists concluded that every 5 g of dietary fiber consumed daily reduced the chances of developing colorectal cancer by about 9%.[11]

However, unlimited intake of soluble dietary fiber may not be prudent.[12] Foods rich in soluble dietary fiber often contain compounds that prevent the digestion of dietary fat. Although this may seem appealing to some individuals who experience difficulty maintaining a healthy body weight, it is unhealthy and may decrease the absorption of essential fatty acids and fat-soluble vitamins. Similarly, soluble fiber intakes greater than 50 g/day may inhibit the digestion of dietary sugars – again, potentially attractive to the overweight but unhealthy. Increasing the amount of simple sugars and starches, such as corn starch, rice starch and potato starch that reaches the colon encourages the microbes to produce lactic acid, not butyrate. While the lack of butyrate produced may be directly unhealthy for the colon, the increased amounts of sugars and starches may also promote the growth of unhealthy bacteria and yeast, adversely affecting the healthy balance of bacterial flora in the guts. Maintaining a balanced amount of dietary fiber intake is thus necessary to obtain its benefits.

Colon Ecology

The colon is a dynamic ecologic system in which human colon cells and immune cells, microbes and ingested foods interact in the near-absence of oxygen. The human gastrointestinal tract normally contains trillions[14] of living bacteria, representing over 400 individual species. Most live in the colon. The goal of dietary maintenance of colon health is to foster a symbiotic relationship, with the human host and its microbial guests living in harmony and balance.

The colon harbors a large variety of microorganisms. The most common bacterial species in the healthy human colon are the *Bifidobacteria* and *Lactobacilli*. In addition, even the healthy colon normally contains pockets of *Clostridia*, yeasts and protozoa. The species of bacteria that most quickly and efficiently produce butyrate in the human colon, and which therefore are the most beneficial and the most desirable, are the *Bifidobacteria* and *Lactobacilli*.

Beneficial Probiotic Organisms

The *Bifidobacteria* are the most common microorganisms in the healthy human digestive tract and are the predominant microbes in human breast milk. *Bifidobacteria* comprise about 50% of all intestinal microflora in the healthy colon and ferment dietary fiber to short chain fatty acids, especially butyrate. By producing large amounts of butyrate, the *Bifidobacteria* support the health and function of human colon cells. In addition, the *Bifidobacteria* suppress the growth of harmful bacteria by keeping the acidity of the colon interior just high enough to inhibit bacterial growth but not too high to affect the colon cells. *Bifidobacteria* also compete with unhealthy bacteria for space within the colon.

Lactobacilli (the "lactic acid bacteria") comprise about 25% of all intestinal microflora. The *Lactobacilli* perform many of the same colon-friendly functions as the *Bifidobacteria* but produce a little more lactic acid, helping the *Bifidobacteria* keep the colon slightly acidic. The *Lactobacilli* also secrete an enzyme that breaks down lactose from milk.[13]

Species of *Saccharomyces*, a yeast commonly living in both the small and large intestines, help stimulate intestinal digestive activities. In addition, they are antagonistic to *Candida albicans* and keep them at bay. These yeasts also enhance immunity in the gut and dietary supplementation with *Saccharomyces boulardii* has been found to support the consistency of healthy bowel movements.[14]

The most common and beneficial bacteria and yeasts share an important fundamental characteristic. They all prefer to feast on soluble dietary fiber. Feed them

> *"The colon is a dynamic system. Its health is directly influenced by our dietary choices."*

and they will produce all the butyrate your colon can eat. Starve them and risk the health of your colon.

Disturbances of Colon Ecology

The colon is a dynamic system. Its health is directly influenced by our dietary choices. These choices impact the supply of nutrition to the gut bacteria and our intestinal cells. A number of common dietary and medical practices can disturb the symbiotic relationship between microorganisms and human cells that is absolutely vital to the health of the colon. Among these are infant formula feeding, low fiber diets, and oral antibiotic therapy.

Infant Formula Feeding — The human gastrointestinal tract is sterile at birth. During birth, the tract is seeded initially by organisms living in the maternal vagina. During breastfeeding, mammary gland microflora contribute the early populations of *Bifidobacteria* that begin to populate the infant's colon. Foodborne microflora and self-inoculation also contribute to early intestinal ecology. Species distribution in the newborn digestive tract is modulated for the first few days of life by maternal antibodies transferred in colostrum. In breastfed infants, over 90% of intestinal bacteria consist of *Bifidobacterium infantis*. In contrast, the intestinal tracts of infants who are not breastfed are characterized by low numbers of *Bifidobacteria* and *Lactobacilli* and high numbers of less healthy *Enterococci*, Coliforms and *Clostridia*. The lack of proper healthy gut bacterial species in childhood has been associated with a number of digestive health issues.[14]

Low Fiber Diets — Lack of dietary fiber for fermentation reduces the supply of butyrate available to colon cells and interferes with their ability to seal the colon off from the bloodstream, increasing the likelihood of toxins and bacteria from the guts entering circulation. As discussed above, butyrate starvation also slows the renewal of colon cells. Insufficient amounts of nonfermentable fiber slows the rate of passage of the digesta, increasing the time available for water absorption by colon cells and providing increased exposure of the longer-lived colon cells to free radicals.[15] Increased water absorption results in stool hardness and affects the consistency of bowel movements.[16] Fiber provides the food for intestinal bacteria and the bulk for optimal bowel function.

Oral Antibiotic Therapy — Antibiotics can also kill beneficial *Lactobacilli* and *Bifidobacteria*. As the numbers of these beneficial bacteria decrease, there is a compensatory increase in the unhealthy species that have been kept under control by the beneficial bacteria, resulting in disturbances in gut ecology. This shift in microbial populations can have a severe impact on colon health. Most importantly, this disturbance of gut ecology may lead to decreased levels of butyrate as most of the overgrown microbial species are inefficient fermenters of dietary fiber. The combination of reduced ability to seal off the colon and increased populations of unhealthy organisms can compromise the colon lining and affect immune function.

Supplemental Prebiotics and Probiotics

The colon is dependent on its microbial residents for nourishment and defense. In turn, our microbes need to eat foods that are healthy for them. Ideally, good food sources of fiber would have been a major part of our diet all of our life, and our colon and its residents would require very little attention from us. Realistically, the average American is fiber deficient and has a colon to reflect it. Restoring the healthy ecological balance in the colon is absolutely mandatory if health and healthy aging are your objectives.

Prebiotics — Starter Foods for Your Microbes

Prebiotics are dietary ingredients often consumed in the form of foods and dietary supplements that stimulate the growth of

> *"Restoring the healthy ecological balance in the colon is absolutely mandatory if health and healthy aging are your objectives."*

Bifidobacteria and *Lactobacilli* species and foster the production of butyrate within the colon. The most widely available prebiotics are fructans (fructooligosaccharides; FOS), inulin and the oligofructoses, galactooligosaccharide and the levans (occurring in tubers and grasses). Foods that contain large amounts of these prebiotics include wheat, onions, asparagus, chicory, banana and artichokes.

These compounds all are indigestible by humans within the small intestine, are converted to short chain fatty acids in the colon and are essentially calorie-free. Fructooligosaccharides (FOS) – These long-chain indigestible sugars are specifically fermented to short-chain fatty acids (especially butyrate) by *Bifidobacteria*. The results of a study published recently in the *Nutrition Journal* confirm that the daily consumption of as little as 2.5 g of FOS increases the proportion of *Bifidobacteria* in the colon.[17] The consumption of FOS by infants has been documented to be safe and to decrease the incidence of infant emesis and regurgitation. In addition to fostering colon health, the products of FOS fermentation may promote cardiovascular health.

Probiotics — Dietary Supplements to Repopulate Your Colon

Probiotics have been defined as oral dietary supplements containing live microbes that enhance colon health. When effective, such supplements increase the numbers of intestinal *Bifidobacteria* and *Lactobacilli* and decrease the numbers of those microbial species that do not produce butyrate. An ideal probiotic supplement will have the following characteristics: 1) The bacteria must survive passage through the stomach and small intestine so that they reach the colon while still alive, 2) They must produce short-chain fatty acids from dietary fiber while in the colon, 3) They must maintain a slightly acidic colonic pH, and 4) They must be capable of eventually permanently repopulating the colon themselves or stimulate other healthy bacterial species to do so.

As suggested by the results of a recently published study, successful reseeding of the colon's microbial populations can support increased immune defenses.[18] According to articles published recently in *Gut* and the *American Journal of Physiology*, this benefit may result from an effect of the probiotic organisms leading to an increase in the stimulation and vigilance of the immune cells that are interspersed within the lining of the colon.[19,20]

Successful reseeding with probiotic species requires at least 6 months of daily ingestion of at least 10 billion "colony forming units" (10^{10} CFU) per species. Successful reseeding may not be possible in some individuals with chronically compromised colon health; they may well require life-long daily supplementation in order to maintain appropriate microbial populations in their colon.

Bacillus coagulans: A Novel, Unique Probiotic Organism

Bacillus coagulans is a bacterial species that may offer unique benefits to digestive health. This bacterium is a spore former and is especially hardy with respect to different intestinal environments. A specific strain of *Bacillus coagulans* known as BC30™ is available as a dietary supplement for digestive health. Research indicates that this particular strain has beneficial immune effects while it also enhances the repopulation of the digestive tract with other friendly bacterial strains. While BC30™ is a transient organism in that it does not colonize the digestive tract itself, it promotes optimal gut ecology and aids in crowding out other non-beneficial organisms.

BC30™ can be an effective nutritional tool on its own or in combination with other

"... a large body of scientific evidence demonstrates conclusively that dietary supplementation with prebiotic/probiotic combinations consistently yields health benefits that extend beyond digestive wellness on several fronts."

multi-strain probiotic dietary supplements to support digestive tract wellness. Since BC30™ is a spore former and is a hardy strain of bacteria, it does not need to be refrigerated.

Combinations of Prebiotics and Probiotics

Because probiotics are the bacteria you want to live in your colon and prebiotics are the food they love best, it would make sense to combine the two, so that you can be sure that the newly-arriving residents have plenty to eat after their trip through your digestive tract. The benefits of "combination supplementation" are well-documented.

The published human clinical trials have been summarized recently in the *Journal of Bioscience and Bioengineering* and the *World Journal of Gastroenterology*.[14,21] This large body of scientific evidence demonstrates conclusively that dietary supplementation with prebiotic/probiotic combinations consistently yields health benefits that extend beyond digestive wellness on several fronts. A review article published recently in the *World Journal of Gastroenterology* recommended *Lactobacillus*-containing "combination supplements" for enhancing digestion of lactose.[22] Conversely, because it encourages normal water management by colon cells and healthy contractions by colonic smooth muscles, "combination supplementation" also promotes the consistency of healthy bowel movements.[21,23]

The Bottom Line

Maintaining healthy digestive function consists of supporting multiple aspects of the complicated physiological function of the gastrointestinal system. While the process of digestion itself is complex, supporting several fundamental aspects of the process can lead to tangible benefits for overall health. Dietary factors are critical as the foundation for digestive health. This entails consuming foods that are healthy and eating an adequate amount of dietary fiber. Nutritional interventions are also a key element. These include supplemental enzymes, fiber supplements, prebiotics and probiotics. An optimally functioning digestive system can yield dividends that can lead to a lifetime of health and wellness.

14

Managing the Inflammatory Response – Natural Support

Better Communication is the Key

Inflammation is the body's natural way of defending itself against insults and protecting the integrity of its organs and systems. The complicated inflammatory response usually remains tightly controlled through a voluminous exchange of intercellular messages transmitted via small proteins ("cytokines") that flow between cells, allowing them to coordinate their defensive, demolition and reconstruction activities. Cytokines also provide "reminders" to the cells that produced them.

How each cell responds to a message depends on what type of cell it is. For example, the cytokine, interleukin-1, will stimulate cells in the hypothalamus to generate a fever but will tell cells in the liver to produce other cytokines that instruct cells elsewhere in the body (such as "TNF- ", which stimulates the proliferation of lymphocytes). The large amount of cytokine "cross talk" creates networks of sequential and simultaneous responses throughout the body.

The regulation of the severity, extent and duration of an inflammatory response to a stimulus depends on whether the stimulus is short-term or persistent. Under normal healthy circumstances the initial inflammatory response will be effective in removing the stimulus and a set of anti-inflammatory cytokines will communicate a "job well done – time to relax" message that will restore the balance between active responses, vigilant surveillance and inactivity in the immune system.

Unfortunately, the complex communication network can become short-circuited or fail. When that happens, either the body may fail to respond effectively to an inflammatory stimulus or it may overreact. As demonstrated in an article published recently in *Blood*, predisposition to inflammatory overreaction increases with age.[1]

As the balance between the pro-inflammatory system and the anti-inflammatory system gradually tips in favor of increased (and possibly excessive) reactivity, the need for effective nutritional support of your immune system becomes increasingly urgent.

Tips for Promoting a Normal Healthy, Balanced Inflammatory Response

Less Heat, More Nutrition

As discussed recently in the *Annals of the New York Academy of Sciences* excessive sugars in the blood can attach abnormally to proteins.[2] In most cases, this sugar-protein combination cannot function properly and in fact is seen by the immune system as foreign. Within the body, these complexes can provoke inflammatory responses in the gums, joints, blood vessels – creating conditions that can impair the health of many tissues and organs.

Cooking foods at high temperatures also generates these complexes that enter your bloodstream after you have eaten the food. Broiled and fried meats and cooked animal fats contain the highest levels. In contrast, fruits and vegetables contain almost none. Replacing some of the pro-inflammatory foods with those that are anti-inflammatory can improve the balance.

Help Your Blood Vessels Help Themselves!

During their travels through your bloodstream, fats can become oxidized by a number of other circulating compounds, including things from the diet. Oxidized fats are potentially dangerous oxidizers of other compounds. Special antioxidants ("paraoxonases") made within immune cells diffuse the danger posed by the oxidized fats in the bloodstream. However, this system can be overwhelmed. If too many of these fat cells collect in one spot, they may trigger a reaction that can throw off the balance of the entire inflammatory system.

Cutting-edge research has shown a clear connection between the amount of fat you eat and an increase in the imbalanced inflammatory response. Research just published in *Nutrition* has documented a direct relationship between dietary fat intake and this imbalanced inflammatory response.[3] The culprit is high levels of dietary saturated fats. So for the sake of your hard-working vascular system – CUT: 1) cut back on red meats and replace them with fresh vegetables and white meats; 2) when you do eat red meat, cut off the fat you can see before cooking (if you don't eat it, it can't hurt you); and 3) cut down the cooking temperature – overcooking red meats just makes them even more harmful.

Antioxidant Vitamins and Nutrients Normalize the Inflammatory Response

Vitamin C and vitamin E inhibit the oxidation of fats in the blood and stimulate the immune system to remove them from the circulation. These actions both protect the cardiovascular system and decrease the body's overall inflammatory "tone."[4] In a study published in the *Journal of Nutrition*, it was found that the amount of vitamin C and E that older men and women consume is proportional to the amounts of fruit and vegetables they eat[5] – eat more fruit and vegetables, eat more vitamins. But if you cannot eat enough fruits and vegetables every day, add supplements containing vitamins C and E to your daily diet.

The antioxidant N-acetylcysteine also supports normalization of the inflammatory response in tissues.[3,6] The findings of a published study demonstrate conclusively that because N-acetylcysteine can enter all cells it is a very effective and efficient antioxidant and supports a healthy inflammatory state throughout the body.[7]

Other powerful dietary antioxidants obtained from fruits and vegetables, such as the flavonoid quercetin and the stilbene resveratrol, also help the immune system support and maintain a healthy cardiovascular system. In addition, research in humans showed that pomegranate juice tones down and helps to stabilize levels of inflammation throughout the cardiovascular system.[8] Nutritional science provides convincing evidence that in addition to beneficial dietary supplements, you can promote a healthy balance in your immune system by adding more fruits and vegetables to your diet.

Don't Forget the Fish (and Fish Oil)

Month after month another study is published that confirms again the lesson of previous studies: fish oils (and the fish that contain them) are powerful promoters of balance in the human immune system. Recently, researchers confirmed that maintaining a healthy inflammatory state depends upon adequate daily consumption

> "Fish oils are powerful promoters of balance in the human immune system."

of fish oils – especially fish oils that are highly refined to contain concentrated levels of the essential fats DHA and EPA, and less fishy contaminants, mercury, pollutants and carcinogens.[9]

Selenium and the Colorful Carotenoids

The mineral selenium and the colorful phytonutrients known as the carotenoids (especially β-carotene, lutein, lycopene, zeaxanthin and β-cryptoxanthin) are powerful antioxidants that help regulate the normal inflammatory response. Research shows that higher selenium and carotenoids consumption promotes health and longevity. This conclusion is verified by the results of a study published recently in the *Journal of Nutrition* showing that subjects with the higher concentrations of selenium and carotenoids in their bodies tended to live the longest.[10]

Pycnogenol® for Immune Support

The powerful patented extract of French maritime pine tree bark, Pycnogenol®, can also help your immune system maintain its balance. For example, in research published recently in *Biomedicine and Pharmacotherapy*, dietary supplementation with Pycnogenol® was shown to inhibit the effects of proinflammatory and pro-aging enzymes, thereby promoting a normal state of inflammatory activity.[11]

Move It and Just Keep on Moving It

The results of the Health, Aging and Body Composition Study, published in the *Journal of the American Geriatrics Society* show quite clearly that <u>one of the most effective things you can do to promote the health of your immune system and maintain inflammatory balance is to perform some combination of physical activities for at least 3 hours every week.</u>[7] Gardening, yard work, housework, walking up and down stairs, walking at least a mile, calisthenics, using small or large weights, bicycle riding or any other activity that requires putting your body in motion all contribute to the production of physiological responses that reduce the "inflammatory tone" of your body.

Stop Smoking!

Smoking is one of the worst activities you can continue to do and still hope to normalize the body's inflammatory response. In addition to contributing to the development of several chronic diseases, smoking leads to a generalized state of inflammation throughout the body. Smoking increases blood levels of inflammatory markers, triggering injury to the vasculature and leading directly to the development of cardiovascular disease. Numerous chemicals associated with cigarette smoke are carcinogens and therefore contribute to the development of several cancers.[12] If you're still smoking, quit! It's the best thing you can do for your health.

15

Sleep – Vital to Health and Healing

Sleep is something we often take for granted. Many of us rarely give it a second thought. However, adequate sleep is crucial to human functionality. Besides providing down-time for the body to heal, it relieves stress and helps the body rejuvenate from the rigors and challenges of our daily lives. Beyond rejuvenating the body, sleep is also necessary for rejuvenating the mind - a tonic for our physical and mental wellness.

With age, our sleep quality normally tends to decline. In fact, a common complaint voiced by many older people is the declining duration of sleep as they reach and live through middle-age. It is well-documented that over the age of 50, added to the shortage of time caused by the demands of family, job, travel, shopping and other obligations, men and women experience a naturally-reduced ability to fall asleep, the sleep they get is shallower and of shorter duration, and they are awakened more easily. Lack of sufficient quality sleep will impair mental focus and decrease the quality of life.

"Lack of sufficient quality sleep will impair mental focus and decrease the quality of life."

Sleep and Cardiovascular Function

There's an even more serious danger lurking under the bed – according to the results of recently published research, routinely getting only 5 hours or less of quality sleep at night is known to double your risk of developing (or exacerbating) high blood pressure.[1] Even *worse* – failing to get at least 7 hours of sleep significantly increases your chances of suffering a heart attack![2] While these studies highlight problems associated with chronic sleep issues, the occasional inability to fall asleep can also be of concern.

Your Third Eye, Melatonin and Sleep

The pineal gland (the historical "third eye"), once thought to possess magical, supernatural or psychic powers, is now known to control daily body rhythms ("chronobiology") in conjunction with light/dark information supplied by the eyes. The major output of the pineal gland is melatonin, a compound made from L-tryptophan and named for its ability to "trick" skin melanocytes (the cells that normally darken upon exposure to sunlight) into lightening their color as if they had never been exposed to light.

Although melatonin has critical functions in the regulation of many circadian (day/night) and seasonal cycles in human physiology and neurobiology, it is best known (and most studied) for its roles in the control of the sleep/wake cycle.

Pineal secretion of melatonin is linked to the *absence* of daylight – bright light triggers the transmission of electrical signals from the retina along a special nerve to the brain's central circadian pacemaker area in the hypothalamus. Because these signals suppress brain secretion of the hormone (norepinephrine) that activates melatonin secretion, lack of bright light (dim light or darkness) allows norepinephrine release by the hypothalamus; in turn, melatonin secretion is activated (in response to *lack* of light).

In most people, melatonin secretion begins about 2 to 4 hours after sunset and ends about 1 to 3 hours after dawn. The amount of melatonin secreted overnight depends on the length of time the retina remains unstimulated by light.

Melatonin Secretion with Age

Like so many other bodily functions, melatonin secretion at night typically declines during middle age. In fact, older men and women who secrete the least melatonin overnight tend to have the most difficulty falling asleep. In addition, older men and women tend to become sleepier earlier in the evening and to awaken earlier in the morning, without changes in the cyclic timing of melatonin secretion – almost as if their brains have learned to anticipate the switching on and off of daylight.

Natural Methods to Enhance Sleep

Melatonin to the Rescue

A little manipulation of your melatonin cycle can go a long way toward restoring a more youthful sleep pattern. A number of gold standard, "randomized placebo-controlled" human clinical trials have shown that the consumption of small amounts of melatonin (0.3 mg to 5 mg) about one hour before bedtime can shorten the time it takes you to fall asleep, can increase the actual amount of time you sleep while also increasing the relative percentage of the time you spend in bed at night during which you are asleep, and reduce "morning after" daytime sleepiness.

The results of a study published recently in the *Journal of Physiology* demonstrate that even "normal" sleepers can enjoy an increased quality of sleep and awaken more refreshed following the consumption of 1.5 mg of melatonin before bedtime.[3] In fact, many folks find that 1 mg of melatonin about a half hour before going to bed does the trick just fine.

Melatonin enhances normal sleep and may improve occasional sleeplessness. This nutrient also has other potentially beneficial effects in the human body. The latest research findings suggest that melatonin can extend maximum lifespan in mice by up to 15% – an effect called "geroprotection." How does melatonin do this?

Free Radical Theory of Aging

According to the free radical theory of aging, the normal oxidative reactions of metabolism that occur in all cells generate free radical electrons which can damage DNA, proteins and cell membranes, resulting in "aging" on the cellular level. Over time, as the number of individual cells that are experiencing "aging" increases, the entire body begins to show signs of the accumulation of damaged cells and proteins – "aging" in its more common sense.

It has long been known that melatonin is a scavenger of free radical electrons, as many studies have confirmed the ability of melatonin to protect DNA and membrane lipids from oxidative damage. Inside cells, melatonin stimulates the synthesis of glutathione (another antioxidant) while inhibiting the activity of oxidizing enzymes such as nitric oxide synthetase and lipoxygenase. A beneficial consequence of melatonin's antioxidant actions is increased stability of membranes both inside and surrounding cells.

Melatonin doesn't just help the body remove free radical electrons after they are formed – it also increases the efficiency of the metabolic reactions that produce free radical electrons, preventing the generation of free radicals in the first place. Melatonin may be even better at this than either vitamin C or vitamin E and in recent research published in the *Journal of Neural Transmission* melatonin was called "the premier molecule to protect cells from oxidative stress."[4] In short, melatonin lowers oxidative stress levels by slowing free radical production, stimulating the body's natural antioxidant defense systems and itself capturing and deactivating free radicals.

Melatonin continues to promote antioxidant effects on the body even after it has been used up. When melatonin captures and deactivates a free radical electron, the melatonin molecule becomes changed into "secondary metabolites" that are as effective as the original melatonin molecule in capturing and deactivating free radical electrons – packing each individual melatonin molecule with plenty of excess capacity for protection against oxidative stress.

Additionally, melatonin is a strong supporter of a healthy and effective immune system. This simple compound is produced by the cells of the immune system and enhances cell-to-cell communication to ensure that challenges to the immune system are met quickly and efficiently.

Thus, in addition to restoring youthful sleep, melatonin can benefit our bodies as a strong antioxidant and immune system stimulant, supporting healthy aging in numerous ways.

Does Eating Sugar Make You Sleepy or Alert?

Athletes used to eat sugary foods just before a competition in the belief that this would increase their performance. However, according to research published recently in the *Journal of Cellular and Molecular Medicine*, a rise in blood sugar concentrations may actually translate into physiological responses that ultimately will reduce wakefulness.[5]

Acutely elevated blood glucose concentrations (as occur after a carbohydrate-rich meal) suppress the secretion of chemicals called orexins (also called hypocretins) by the hypothalamus. One of the major functions of these chemicals is to prevent the pineal gland from secreting melatonin. By suppressing melatonin secretion, they may enhance wakefulness. However, since elevated blood sugar suppresses the release of orexins, melatonin secretion is increased, causing a sense of drowsiness. Fasting may have just the opposite effect. As blood glucose concentrations decline, the mind becomes more alert.[5]

L-Tryptophan as a Natural Sleep Promoter

Modern nutritional mythology holds that eating turkey meat will make you sleepy because it is a rich source of the amino acid, L-tryptophan. The validity of this legend is under debate by nutritionists. However, because melatonin is made from L-tryptophan in the pineal gland, it makes sense that L-tryptophan could contribute to increasing melatonin secretion and thus help relieve occasional sleeplessness.

This possibility was tested in a study published recently in the *American Journal of Clinical Nutrition*.[6] These researchers discovered that dietary supplementation with a single "dose" of 2 g (2000 mg) of L-tryptophan in the evening reduced sleepiness the next morning and improved the ability to concentrate in healthy adults.

Valerian – A Relaxing Herb

Extracts of the roots of valerian (*Valeriana officinalis*) contain volatile oils that, according to the German Commission E, can support normalization of "restlessness and nervous disturbance of sleep." In human studies, 450 mg to 1200 mg of oral valerian root extract in the evening have shortened the time to fall asleep, improved the quality of sleep and decreased daytime drowsiness for adults with difficulty sleeping. The results of a study published recently in *Molecular Brain Research* show that compounds in valerian root extract stimulate the sleep-inducing areas of the brain and enhance normal sleep.[7] The amount of extract consumed is important; more than 400 mg was required to improve sleep quality. Timing also is important; valerian too close to bedtime may not allow enough time for absorption before sleep is attempted.

Green Tea for Relaxation

The amino acid L-theanine is unique to tea leaves and is primarily obtained in the diet by drinking green tea. Studies in rats and humans have demonstrated that the consumption of L-theanine increases the release of dopamine and serotonin in the brain and increases brain alpha-wave activity, a sign of relaxation and increasing calmness. Research suggests that the consumption of 200 mg of L-theanine about one hour before bedtime can help one relax, which may enhance the ability to sleep.

Volatile Oils to Support Healthy Sleep

In a placebo-controlled experiment published recently in *Chronobiology International*, exposure of adult men and women to the scent of lavender volatile oils at bedtime significantly increased sleep duration, the percentage of sleep spent in deep sleep and subjects' self-reported morning vigor.[8] In contrast, the results of another placebo-controlled experiment published recently in *Biological Psychology* indicate that exposure to the scent of peppermint volatile oils increases alertness and inhibits sleep.[9] Together, these research findings suggest that the scent of some relaxing volatile oils can help normalize sleep patterns while simultaneously pleasing the senses.

Sleep for Vitality and Vigor

Sleep is an essential practice for health and the lack of sleep has adverse effects on normal well-being. By promoting healthy sleep patterns through lifestyle practices and dietary supplementation, one is able to increase vitality, normalize stress and refresh our body's ability to cope with the rigors of daily life.

16

Prostate Health: Nutritional Support for Healthy Function

The prostate is a walnut sized gland that is a part of the male reproductive system located in the pelvic area. The prostate stores and produces seminal fluid, which serves as nourishment for the sperm. As men age, the prostate can often be an area of concern. Diverse conditions can affect the prostate and impact sexual function as well as normal urination. Because these functions are important for wellness, supporting healthy prostate gland function becomes a priority for men as they age.

The key to promoting prostate health is to ensure the nourishment and proper functioning of the cells it is made up of. Ensuring cellular health also ensures that the cellular cycle of growth, reproduction and differentiation occurs normally. The health of the cells is a determining factor for the prostate to maintain its normal size. However, it is difficult to know how healthy these cells are. In fact, the ability of cells to grow and differentiate normally can already have been lost even if the prostate appears normal in size.

As mentioned above, every approach to supporting and promoting the health and stability of the prostate gland is based on helping the cells of the gland control their normal life cycle. A proper rate of replacement of old cells with new will allow the gland to retain its normal size, shape and functions. Fortunately, a virtual cornucopia of nutritional factors help prostate gland cells retain tight control over the timing of their life cycles and strictly regulate their reproductive rate. Used wisely, the nutritional support that is available today can help keep any man's prostate healthy with age.

> *"Every approach to supporting and promoting the health and stability of the prostate gland is based on helping the cells of the gland control their normal life cycle."*

A Nutritional Armamentarium for Prostate Health

Lycopene

Lycopene, a carotenoid phytonutrient most abundant in tomatoes and pink grapefruit, contributes to the maintenance of normal healthy human prostate tissues and helps prostate gland cells control their reproductive rate by acting as an antioxidant to protect cellular DNA from oxidation. The beneficial effects of lycopene on the prostate are substantiated by the results of human studies that suggest that prostate health can be enhanced by the routine daily consumption of at least 6.5 mg of lycopene.[1]

Tomatoes

Every time the link between tomatoes and prostate health is examined, the answer is the same – eating at least one tomato, or at least one serving of tomato sauce in any form, at least once a day is a superb and effective way to keep your prostate healthy. The US Food and Drug Administration agrees and announced on November 8, 2005, that "very limited and preliminary scientific research suggests that eating one-half to one cup of tomatoes and/or tomato sauce a week may reduce the risk of prostate cancer."

Selenium

A large body of evidence consistently illustrates the potent prostate-promoting properties of selenium. The strong links between selenium and prostate health were examined in a thorough analysis that was recently published.[2] These scientists concluded that dietary supplementation with selenium increased a man's chances of maintaining a healthy prostate by about 40%. According to other research selenium benefits the prostate by honing in on prostate cells and directly helping them maintain a healthy life cycle and lifestyle.[3,4]

The US Food and Drug Administration agrees that selenium is good for the prostate and announced on February 21, 2003, that "Selenium may reduce the risk of certain cancers. Some scientific evidence suggests that consumption of selenium may reduce the risk of certain forms of cancer" and "Selenium may produce anticarcinogenic effects in the body. Some scientific evidence suggests that consumption of selenium may produce anticarcinogenic effects in the body."

Vitamin E

Scientific evidence reported recently confirms that dietary supplementation with vitamin E helps to protect the human prostate gland by promotion of the prostate cell's own internal cell cycle-regulating clock.[5,6,7] By encouraging the cells to function as they are programmed, vitamin E plays an important role in healthy prostate function. Of course, vitamin E is also a strong antioxidant and confers protection in this way.

Lycopene plus Vitamin E

A report published recently in the *Journal of Nutrition* shows that combining vitamin E supplementation with extra lycopene may be even more beneficial than is either nutrient alone[8] – yet another example of nutrients working together to produce greater good than they can individually.

Stinging Nettle (Urtica dioica L.)

The roots of the stinging nettle plant contain antioxidants that are active in the human prostate and may help prostate gland cells maintain population stability.[9,10]

Saw Palmetto

Compounds found in saw palmetto berries have been shown to contribute to the normal stability of cell cycle regulation in prostate gland cells. Human clinical trials have confirmed that dietary supplementation with 320 mg or more of a phytosterol-rich extract of saw palmetto berries is a powerful ally to the prostate gland. In addition, after performing a detailed and very rigorous mathematical analysis of all of the available data on the human responses to daily dietary supplementation with saw palmetto berry extract, the prestigious Cochrane Collaborative Review Group concluded that this extract is a strong promoter of prostate health.[11]

Pomegranate Fruit

The antioxidant strength of the phytonutrients in pomegranate fruit allows this fruit to bolster the regulation of the prostate gland cell cycle. As we have seen, strong antioxidants and cell cycle regulators are beneficial to the prostate gland. Indeed, the results of research published recently in *Cell Cycle* and *Proceedings of the National Academy of Sciences of the* USA demonstrate that pomegranate fruit phytonutrients help human prostate gland cells regulate their life cycles and functions.[12,13]

African Prune Tree (Pygeum africanum)

Research further shows that phytonutrients contained in the bark of the African prune tree, *Pygeum africanum*, are valuable promoters of prostate health. As little as 100 mg daily provide support to prostate cells in their struggle to maintain the stability of their life cycles.[14]

β-Sitosterol

A phytosterol phytonutrient, β-sitosterol closely resembles cholesterol, but has just the right small differences to make it health-promoting instead of health-threatening. Similar to their conclusions regarding saw palmetto berry extract, the prestigious Cochrane Collaborative Review Group has concluded that daily dietary supplementation with β-sitosterol helps the cells of the prostate gland retain and maintain the necessary healthy tight regulation of their cell cycles and rate of cell division and can make an important contribution to the nutritional support of the prostate gland.[15] β–sitosterol can be added to the diet as peanut oil, extra virgin olive oil, sesame oil, soybean oil, raw or roasted peanuts or as a component of a high-quality dietary supplement.

Milk Thistle

Extracts of milk thistle have been associated with health benefits to the liver for many centuries. The 21st century has seen this powerful liver health promoter come into its own as a strong supporter of the prostate gland. Research published recently in *Biomedical Papers* has confirmed the role of the phytonutrients in milk thistle seeds in the maintenance of healthy regulation of the prostate cell cycle and the contribution of these phytonutrients to prostate health.[16]

Zinc

Zinc is a key nutrient that is present in high concentrations in prostate tissue. Recent research results suggest that an abundant supply of zinc in the body may support normal metabolic control in prostate cells, allowing them to maintain regularity of their cellular differentiation cycles.[17]

Resveratrol

Resveratrol, the major bioactive phytonutrient in red grapes supports prostate gland health by helping prostate gland cells maintain synchronized regulation of their life cycles.[18] A high-quality dietary supplement containing resveratrol, may also enhance the body's ability keep your prostate vibrantly healthy.

> "Men who regularly participated in outdoor activities that allowed exposure to sunlight had healthier prostate glands than men who consciously avoided sun exposure."

Get Out Once in a While

Some sunlight is good for you. By increasing your natural production of vitamin D, sunlight contributes to bone health, skin health, brain health, heart health, gut health, breast health, reproductive system health and now – prostate health. According to published research men who regularly participated in outdoor activities that allowed exposure to sunlight had healthier prostate glands than men who consciously avoided sun exposure.[19] Don't hide from the sun – seek the light!

Don't Be Afraid of Calcium

A small "calcium scare" was started a few years ago by a single report that "high" calcium intake might be detrimental to prostate health.[20] However, in that report, a "high" calcium intake was 50% of the RDA. The good news – this false alarm has been contradicted conclusively by the findings of 2 subsequent studies published recently which showed that calcium intake is in fact not detrimental to prostate health.[21,22] Eat your calcium and vitamin D, and get some sun – they're good for you!

Don't Overcook Meat

When meat is cooked at very high temperatures in order to make it "well done" or "very well done" the cooking process generates potentially carcinogenic hydrocarbons within the meat. The results of the Prostate, Lung, Colorectal, and Ovarian Cancer Screening Trial of the US National Cancer Institute, published recently in *Cancer Research* show clearly that eating any overcooked meat, even just once a week, directly harms the human prostate.[23] "Lighten up" your meat and live more happily, longer.

A number of nutritional interventions are available that have strong research supporting their ability to support prostate health. Certain vitamins, minerals and herbs such as saw palmetto and African prune, as well as phytochemicals such as β-sitosterol provide potent options for promoting healthy prostate function and ensuring that prostatic cells are happy and healthy.

17

Stressed Out? - Rejuvenate Your Mind and Body with Adaptogens

The body has a high capacity to adapt to stressful situations that can take various forms. Regardless of the stressors we throw its way, the body has an amazing capacity to react to them and recover normal functionality. However, without the support it needs on a constant basis to overcome stressful situations, even the body can show signs of breakdown, and wear and tear. The effects of chronic stress are well-documented. High levels of constant stress are bad for the body and diminish health. The nature of stressors can be in the form of physical stress or mental and emotional stress. Any of these types of stressors can trigger the body's stress response. The ability of the body to cope with stress determines the level of health in any individual.

> *"The ability of the body to cope with stress determines the level of health in any individual."*

Fight or Flight?

The body's stress response can be divided into three general phases in accordance with the work of the stress researcher Hans Selye. These three phases of the stress response include the alarm phase, the resistance phase, and the exhaustion phase. The *alarm* reaction involves what we know as the *fight or flight* response.

In this acute phase, which is a normal component of the body's stress response, signals from the pituitary gland cause the adrenal glands to release adrenaline and other stress hormones. This allows the body to maintain a high state of vigilance to quickly react to the stressor it is facing. Heart rate increases as blood is circulated to the peripheral tissues in preparation for quick action. The rate of breathing increases and the supply of oxygen to the brain is increased. Blood sugar also increases in response to perceived need by the muscles.

While this initial phase arms the body for the short haul, the second phase of the stress response prepares the body to cope with extended periods of stress, and is known as the *resistance* phase. Cortisol and related hormones of the adrenal cortex are responsible for the physiological effects of this phase. The effects of the cortisol response include the conversion of protein into energy so the body has enough energy stores to cope with the depletion of its glucose supply. Other short-term effects of the resistance phase include providing the body with the emotional strength it needs to cope with stress and enhance it's ability to perform strenuous work, while promoting a strong immune reaction. Cortisol is quite necessary when the body is faced with acute stressors; yet prolonged elevations in cortisol levels, and hence prolonging the resistance phase, can lead to detrimental health effects.

Feeling Tired?

Chronic elevations in cortisol and related stress hormones from the body being under constant stress can lead to the third and final phase of the stress response: *exhaustion*. This is characterized by an inability of the body to deal with the effects of stress and results from the depletion of electrolytes such as potassium. It also results from an inability of the adrenal glands to produce the hormones required to be in this constant state of hypervigilance.

This manifests in weakened organ function and depleted immune function. It also manifests as cellular dysfunction and problems with blood sugar regulation.

The shift of metabolic resources away from daily activities in response to stress predisposes us to a reduced ability to perform "cognitive mental processes" (learning and remembering) and impaired immune defenses. Thus, in order to maintain the body's ability to cope with normal levels of stress, the body requires fundamental support to avoid the consequences of the exhaustion phase of the stress response.

Fundamentals for managing stress include relaxation exercises. These techniques are geared to producing a state of relaxation in the body, which is the opposite of the stress response. While under stress, the sympathetic nervous system is dominant, during relaxation, the parasympathetic nervous system dominates. This is characterized by shunting of blood back from the periphery to the core organs.

Lifestyle Activities that Enhance the Body's Stress Response

Relaxation can be induced through a variety of activities. Meditation and deep breathing exercises are excellent for inducing a state of relaxation of the mind and body. Surprisingly, exercise is also an important component of a stress management program. Acutely, exercise itself induces physical stress on tissues of the body. However, the long-term effects of exercise are to relax the body by strengthening its ability to deal with stress and enhance mood function.

Another important aspect of dealing with stress is mito-chondrial health. The mitochondria in cells are the energy factories where cellular energy production occurs. The production of energy also leads to the production of free radicals. Hence, damage to the mitochondria and to the cells that contain them can occur at a rapid rate. Mitochondrial function has been shown to decrease with age as a result of oxidative stress, predisposing aged individuals to decreased ability to cope with stressful situations and increasing the chances of poor cellular health. Research has shown that resistance exercise restores mitochondrial function in the skeletal muscle of aging individuals, allowing their bodies to better withstand the physical aspects of stress.[1]

Dietary Habits to Reduce the Effects of Stress

Certain dietary habits can interfere with our ability to deal with stress and even increase the effects of stress on the body. Some of these factors are the obvious ones and include excessive alcohol consumption, smoking tobacco products, eating sugar-rich foods and high amounts of simple carbohydrates, skipping meals so the body does not receive adequate nutrition at regular intervals, failing to eat sufficient amounts of high-quality protein to support immune health and blood sugar regulation, and taking in large amounts of stimulants such as caffeine.

On the contrary, a diet high in essential fatty acids, rich in fruits and vegetables that contain important antioxidants, whole grains, and nutrient-rich foods (as opposed to eating empty calories) that contain essential vitamins and minerals all are supportive of the body's stress response. Adding a high-quality, nutritionally complete multivitamin that contains the essential B vitamins, vitamin C and other antioxidant nutrients, such as CoQ10, alpha lipoic acid, and polyphenols, strengthens the foundation of nutritional support necessary for achieving the ability to cope with stressful situations.

Adaptogens – Help You to Adapt

Several herbal remedies can be extremely useful for normalizing the body's stress response. These herbs fall into the category known as adaptogens. Adaptogens increase the ability of the human body to respond ("adapt") to a variety of chemical, biological and physical stressors. A common theme among these rejuvenating tonic herbs is that they are rich in naturally-occurring antioxidants. However, they have properties beyond their antioxidant capabilities that make them restorative of the body's stress-handling ability. Some of the more well-known herbs falling into this category include the various ginsengs, licorice root, eleuthero and ashwagandha. All of these herbs are somewhat similar in nature in that they support the body's natural response to stress. However, they are each somewhat different in terms of the type of situations they are indicated in. They are all superb adaptogens.

Rhodiola rosea - The "Gold-Standard" Adaptogen

Also known as golden root and Arctic root, *Rhodiola rosea* has been shown to have superior adaptogenic properties that support the various phases of the body's stress response. Extracts of *Rhodiola rosea* root contain a variety of active phytonutrients (flavonoids); the best known are salidroside (also called rhodioloside or rhodosin), rodiolin, rosin, rosavin, rosarin, rosaridin and p-tyrosol.

> "In experiments in animals, Rhodiola rosea root extract has been found to improve physical working capacity by increasing the efficiency of conversion of nutrients into energy in muscle cells during exhaustive work."

Rhodiola rosea Enhances Physical Performance

Scandinavian and Russian professional and Olympic athletes have supplemented with *Rhodiola rosea* root extract for years to maximize endurance and accelerate muscle cell recovery after exercise. According to a detailed summary of research conducted within the former Soviet Union on *Rhodiola rosea* root extract, daily consumption of 200 to 600 mg of this herbal preparation has been relied upon for its abilities to 1) sustain a high level of conversion of energy to work during strenuous exercise; 2) reduce the recovery time immediately after a strenuous event; and 3) stimulate protein deposition and muscle growth.[2] Although it is not possible to confirm this author's evaluation of the research (available only in the original Russian), there is some independent scientific evidence that supports the ability of *Rhodiola rosea* root extract to support performance under stress.

In experiments in animals, *Rhodiola rosea* root extract has been found to improve physical working capacity by increasing the efficiency of conversion of nutrients into energy in muscle cells during exhaustive work. This effect of *Rhodiola rosea* root extract on muscle cells can explain at least in part the demonstration, published in the *International Journal of Sport Nutrition and Exercise Metabolism*, that compared to the lack of effects of placebo, the consumption of 200 mg of *Rhodiola rosea* root extract (standardized to 3% rosavin + 1% salidroside) one hour before testing produced increased endurance (time to exhaustion) and maximum oxygen delivery during exercise without an increase in work by the lungs.[3] In another experiment, untrained volunteers who consumed *Rhodiola rosea* root extract prior to beginning controlled exercise experienced faster recovery of muscle function and less soreness when they became exhausted.

Together, this body of science suggests that the capacity to perform any activity, even the activities of daily work, can be sustained and supported by appropriately timed dietary supplementation with *Rhodiola rosea* root extract.

Rhodiola rosea Promotes Mental Performance

Rhodiola rosea root flavonoids enjoy a reputation for stimulating the nervous system, increasing the ability to concentrate, enhancing the quality of work performance, enhancing healthy sleep and eliminating tiredness. For example, the flavonoids in these roots were shown to decrease mental fatigue and increase physical fitness, associative thinking and short-term memory, ability to perform mathematical calculations, ability to concentrate and ability to perform on standardized tests in studies of students during "exam week" and young physicians during generally stressful night shifts. It is likely that, as with muscular work, *Rhodiola rosea* root extract enhances the efficiency of physiological energy generation, and thus supports efficient mental function even during periods of energy-draining physical and mental stress.

Rhodiola rosea Strengthens Immune System Performance

According to recently published research, the flavonoids in *Rhodiola rosea* roots are effective promoters of the innate response of the immune system.[4] Further studies suggest that Rhodiola enhances the production of several chemical messengers of the immune system that function as proliferators of a highly vigilant immune response.[5] Chinese researchers studying the immune modulating effects of Rhodiola have also concluded that the herb has modulatory effects on both the Th1 and Th2 response of the human immune system, thus showing an ability to beneficially balance the immune response.[6] Through its influence on cytokine and immune protein expression, Rhodiola may promote an active, healthy immune response.

Rhodiola rosea may be an ideal adaptogenic herb that is able to support the human stress response by relieving feelings of tiredness and lethargy, by tonifying the body to increase work capacity and physical endurance, by enhancing cognitive function through its ability to support concentration and memory, and by modulating immune function to promote an enhanced immune response.

18

Liver Health: Support the Body's Detox System

Liver Function

Your liver is your body's own Environmental Protection Agency – it works continuously to screen, monitor and cleanse the contents of your blood – quite an important job! The ability of your liver to perform its cleansing operations efficiently and effectively depends on the balance between its cleansing capacity, the amount of cleansing you ask it to perform and the tools you provide to help it perform its functions.

The Liver Needs Help

While the liver is an extremely efficient organ, it can be overwhelmed with toxins that accumulate as a result of lifestyle activities. Things that can contribute to the pool of toxins that the liver must detoxify include the foods we eat, the air we breathe, and the liquids we drink. Other contributors to the overall toxic burden include drugs, heavy metals, and other chemicals we are exposed to at work and home. Smoking and alcohol intake are also obvious contributors to our overall toxic load. All of these factors play a part in increasing the liver's workload. If liver supportive cofactors are not present in adequate amounts, the liver can become inefficient at performing its duties. Cofactors necessary for liver health and function include antioxidants present in fruits and vegetables, which function to help the liver directly and support our body's production of innate antioxidants that fortify the liver's detoxifying capacity. Thus, in order to fully support liver function, dietary and lifestyle factors that enhance liver health must be implemented.

Published research shows that dietary factors can make a large contribution to the liver's overall efficiency – for example, in an animal study published in *Biomedical Research*, drinking green tea (which has a high content of catechins such as EGCG) helped protect rat livers from the damage caused by a deadly hepatotoxin.[1] Another study in rats recently published in the *World Journal of Gastroenterology* showed that the dietary supplement N-acetylcysteine helps the liver protect itself.[2] In yet another study published in the *Journal of Nutrition*, adding fish oil supplements to the human diet was found to accelerate the removal of some detoxified toxins from the liver.[3] In contrast, the consumption of alcoholic beverages was again shown to interfere with human liver function in a recently published study.[4]

> "In order to fully support liver function, dietary and lifestyle factors that enhance liver health must be implemented."

The liver is a complex factory that requires many individual tools and materials to foster the efficient performance of its machinery. Some of these tools perform very specialized functions while others are generally useful to the entire organ. You can assist your liver by providing the tools and help it needs. On the other hand, you have the ability to prevent your liver from doing its array of jobs effectively. Recognizing the balance between help and harm will enable your liver to remain healthy for decades, which is a vital component to healthy longevity.

Lifestyle Choices that Keep Your Liver from Getting Old

Eat, Don't Cook

Many of the biochemical processes that the liver must perform in order to help you stay healthy require the presence of vitamins, minerals and phytonutrients that are most abundant in the vegetables and fruit that you eat. Including these foods in your daily diet will keep your liver cells fully prepared for the challenges that the rest of your diet and body will provide. However, the activity of many of the vitamins and other nutrients present in the diet is decreased by cooking. As explained in a recent review article, cooking vegetables (except beans and potatoes) destroys many of the nutrients the liver craves.[5] It is much more efficient (from your liver's point of view) to eat uncooked vegetables and fruit. Thus, adding raw foods to your diet can help increase the efficiency of liver function. High-quality dietary supplementation can also help bridge the gap between supply and demand and can "level off" day-to-day fluctuations in the nutrient and phytonutrient contents of the foods you consume.

Exception: Some foods need to be cooked to maximize the availability of liver-healthy phytonutrients. As an example, tomatoes contain liver-supportive nutrients in their fibrous materials, so they must be cooked to maximize the release of those nutrients for absorption into your blood.

Enjoy the Colors of the Rainbow

No single food contains all of the beneficial liver-enhancing compounds.[6] Interestingly, foods of different natural colors tend to contain greater amounts of different groups of these compounds. The varying and brilliant colors of fruits and vegetables are reflective of their differing polyphenol content. Various polyphenols are liver-supportive because they have antioxidant properties and confer additional health benefits. The truth is that if all of the whole fruits and vegetables you eat are white, or even green, you will be short-changing your poor overworked liver. (You can find charts linking the colors of foods and the nutrients they represent at http://www.5aday.org).[6] Colorful meals are more than just visually pleasing – they are absolutely necessary for keeping your liver from getting old before its time.

> "Colorful meals are more than just visually pleasing – they are absolutely necessary for keeping your liver from getting old before its time."

Enjoy the Spice(s) of Life

In a presentation to the Fourth International Congress on Vegetarian Nutrition, held in Loma Linda, CA, April 8–11, 2002, Dr. Johanna W. Lampe explained that even though they are thought of primarily as adding flavor or aroma to a meal, all of the spices found in the kitchen actually are used by the body to promote health, and many find their happiest home in liver cells, where they provide additional support for the biochemical functions that are required for detoxification.[7] Spices such as turmeric, cinnamon, cardamom, cumin, coriander and saffron are just a handful that are known to enhance liver function. Go beyond salt and pepper and discover the taste delight of the common as well as the rarely used spices. Flavor up your foods and spice up your liver health.

Give Your Liver a Vacation

As we mentioned above, easing your liver's burden by making healthy dietary and lifestyle choices is healthy and beneficial. For your liver's sake, consider reducing its heavy burden by increasing the proportion of your diet that is made up of organically-grown, pesticide- and herbicide-free, preservative-free, additive-free foods. Why intentionally add to the work that must be done by a part of your body that is so very vital to staying healthy throughout many decades of life?

Cut Down on Unhealthy Fats

The more saturated fats and omega-6 polyunsaturated fats (omega-6 PUFA) you eat, the more fat gets deposited in your liver (as well as everywhere else). When the liver stores too much fat, it becomes clogged and much less efficient at detoxifying chemicals and toxins in the blood.

On the other hand, eating healthy fats can help optimize liver function. As shown in recent research published in *Circulation*, omega-3 PUFA (fish oils) are utilized in cell membranes and in anti-inflammatory processes and are not stored in the liver as fat.[8] One way of reducing the stress on your liver is to ease up on animal fat and omega-6 rich vegetable oil consumption on the one hand and to replace the foods that contain them with healthy servings of fatty cold-water fish and olive oil. Supplementing with a high-quality dietary supplement rich in fish oils is also liver-healthy. Shifting the balance of the fats you consume away from saturated fats and omega-6 PUFA and toward omega-3 PUFA can keep your liver smiling during those extra decades of life.

Don't Give Your Liver a Hangover

No alcohol-containing beverage is totally safe and every sip of any amount (large or small) of alcohol challenges your liver's ability to perform several functions quickly and without error. Although every molecule of alcohol processed by your liver means one less that might affect your brain, that molecule of alcohol could work with stored fat to change a healthy liver into an unhealthy one. The risk increases with increasing alcohol consumption. In addition, alcohol is known to stimulate the liver to produce enzymes that can interfere with the metabolism of many medications, reducing their effectiveness. No matter how you look at it, there is no way to conclude that any amount of alcohol is healthy for your liver. The less you drink, the more your liver will thank you and continue performing at its best for decades.

Don't Overmedicate Your Pain

Several over-the counter and prescription pain medications have well-known liver damaging side effects when used chronically. All of these medications are metabolized by the liver, increasing its metabolic burden and, with excessive use, they may cause the liver harm. As with any other condition, prevention of pain always is preferable to treatment. Controlled exercise, improved posture, chiropractic adjustments and stress reduction, as well as a good night's sleep, can help decrease the need for pain-relieving medications. In addition, a slow-down in the pace of life can help prevent minor accidents with their annoying consequences.

Stop Smoking!

Tobacco smoke contains at least 40 recognized carcinogens that can cause harm to many parts of the body besides the lungs, including the liver. In addition, there are over 2000 separate chemicals in cigarette smoke that are capable of oxidizing cell membranes and proteins. Certainly, nicotine is an addictive drug, much like alcohol. And just as certainly, both alcohol and nicotine are hepatotoxic. No matter what other "protective" steps you may take, continued cigarette smoking will continue to damage your liver and lead to early liver disease.

Support Your Gallbladder along with Your Liver

Fat floats. This is a problem because fats in most of the foods you eat (if not all) cannot pass through your small intestinal lining to reach your blood stream and the rest of your body without first being dissolved in water. Your liver, gallbladder, pancreas and small intestine team up to accomplish this very complicated chemical feat. In its part, your liver passes along to your gallbladder bile acids and bile salts that help fats in your gut dissolve in water, as well as excess cholesterol, fat-soluble vitamins, steroid hormones, and other metabolic wastes that do not otherwise dissolve in water. Some of the materials sent to the gut by the gallbladder are later excreted in the stool. This represents a major pathway for the removal of estrogens, cholesterol and some "detoxified" toxins from the body and is a vital component of health maintenance. As is evident, the gallbladder is a major contributor to the overall detoxification process.

The smooth operation of this system requires the routine production of healthy bile by the liver. Several studies point to dietary and lifestyle measures that can help to promote the efficiency of the gallbladder, lending support to this vital portion of the detoxification system. Papers published in the *Journal of the American Medical Association*, the *American Journal of Epidemiology*, the *Annals of Internal Medicine* and the *American Journal of Clinical Nutrition* have shown that eating peanuts and mixed nuts, and drinking coffee or tea every day, while decreasing animal fat consumption and trimming your waistline, are all factors that can help your gallbladder continue humming along in good health.[9,10,11,12]

Supply Your Liver with the Cofactors It Needs

Most of the machinery your liver cells need to preserve health is generated within liver cells themselves. However, the machinery requires additional tools in order to function at its absolute best. Most of these tools can be obtained from eating healthy foods, especially colorful raw fruits and vegetables. However, our diets are often low in many of the necessary foods and, in some cases, it might take an enormous amount of certain foods everyday to satisfy your liver's needs. In those cases, dietary supplements can allow you to keep your liver fully supplied while still satisfying your food preferences.

Critical Tools for a Healthy Liver

Vitamin C, Vitamin E, Beta-Carotene, Alpha-Lipoic Acid and Selenium

> "...another recently published study confirmed that the liver, bile duct and gallbladder all receive valuable support from the phytonutrients present within green tea."

This group of nutrients forms the foundation of the liver's ability to protect itself from the "collateral damage" that could be caused during the chemical reactions it performs when regulating energy flow to the body, rebalancing amino acids, packaging and repackaging fats and cholesterol, producing bile acids, and converting toxins to harmless compounds. A large body of scientific evidence conclusively demonstrates that each of these nutrients works individually to control free radical production while they cooperate in controlling overall cellular exposure to harmful chemicals.[13] By recycling other antioxidants within liver cells, alpha-lipoic acid increases their efficiency and vastly enhances the antioxidant capacities of vitamin C, vitamin E, selenium and the carotenoids. Because it can function both within the interior of a cell and within its membranes, alpha-lipoic acid is the most versatile of all antioxidants. Alpha-lipoic acid also protects hepatocytes from free radical damage caused by excessive heavy metal exposure. In addition, the antioxidant actions of alpha-lipoic acid serve to normalize the overall inflammatory response.

Green Tea Catechins

One cup of brewed green tea contains about 200 mg of polyphenols, about half of which is (−)-epigallocatechin-3-gallate (EGCG). As shown in a study published in *Biomedical Research*, drinking green tea (which has a high content of catechins) protects the liver from the damage caused by free radicals.[1] The results of another recently published study confirmed that the liver, bile duct and gallbladder all receive valuable support from the phytonutrients present within green tea.[14]

N-Acetylcysteine

After absorption and uptake by the liver, N-acetylcysteine stimulates the synthesis of one of the most important antioxidant compounds within liver cells – glutathione – and, as shown in a study recently published in the *World Journal of Gastroenterology*, N-acetylcysteine promotes the health of liver cells by protecting them against harm.[2]

Fish Oils

Healthy fats, as those found in fish oil, may support the liver's normal metabolic functions. Taking healthy fats also beneficially changes the ratio of healthy fats to unhealthy fats in the diet. Unhealthy fats, as mentioned above, bog down the liver's ability to detoxify harmful chemicals. As reported in a study published in the *Journal of Nutrition*, healthy amounts of fish oil supplements (3000 mg to 5000 mg daily) support fat metabolism in the liver, as well as bile production and liver function.[3] In addition, unlike unhealthy fats, fish oils are not stored within the liver. Replacing sources of other dietary fats with fish oils or fatty fish can further promote liver health.

Milk Thistle (silymarin)

Milk thistle (*Silybum marianum*) was used in classical Greece to support healthy liver and gallbladder function and to protect the liver against toxins. Its active ingredient, silymarin (actually a collection of related compounds found primarily in the seeds), acts to promote healthy liver cell function by stimulating the activity of antioxidant compounds, while itself acting as an antioxidant, stabilizing liver cell membranes and increasing their resistance to penetration by toxins, stimulating the regeneration of normal liver cells and promoting bile production and secretion.

Curcumin (from Turmeric)

Curcuminoids are phytonutrients from turmeric that are responsible for the brilliant orange color of this culinary and medicinal spice. They have tremendous antioxidant properties and have been used for centuries as components of liver-supportive formulas in the Ayurvedic tradition. Several studies, performed in the laboratory and in living organisms, confirm the ability of curcumin to protect the liver against damage caused by hepatotoxic chemicals.[15] It seems that curcumin has the ability to upregulate the function of several antioxidant enzymes, which facilitate protection of liver cells against free radical damage. Studies also show that curcumin activates the essential detoxifying enzyme glutathoine-s-transferase, which facilitates phase II detoxification activities, including conjugation of several chemical compounds with glutathione, leading to their elimination from the body.[16] Being a powerful antioxidant stimulator, curcumin is a useful compound for liver health and function.

Supporting liver function by eating right, limiting alcohol, avoiding tobacco smoke, and providing it the critical nutrients and cofactors it needs to keep functioning at a high level can ensure that it will give you its best effort in keeping you healthy and fit.

19

Brain Health – Maintain a Sharp Mind and Support Cognitive Function

It's obvious to everyone that healthy brain function is essential to life. The brain is the organ that transmits signals to every other organ of the body, coordinating each of their functions with smooth precision. This process is conducted with such regularity that we often take it for granted and don't give it a second thought. However, the brain is also the seat of mental focus and cognitive function. In young age, these faculties work without a hitch. However, as we get older we often notice that we begin to lose a step; our cognitive faculties may not be what they once were and our memory begins to decline. Mental sharpness and clarity, accurate memory and quick decision-making, all communicated clearly and with confidence – this is how our brain used to function. Now, perhaps not so much. Yet, there are things that can help us maintain the cognitive faculties of our youth. By incorporating healthy lifestyle choices and intelligent nutritional management, we can remain sharp far longer than we might have imagined.

Brain Aging

Once past middle-age, the human brain begins a normal decline in performance that is linked to anatomic and biochemical losses. Free radical accumulation over the years takes its toll and begins to affect neural structures and functions. Not only does the number of active brain cells (**neurons**) decline, those that remain may communicate in an increasingly haphazard manner as they "lose touch" with the cells around them and with whom they have enjoyed many years of smooth cooperation. Some neurons actually shrink away from their neighbors, presenting a strong barrier to the cooperation among many neurons that every brain function requires. Neurons also may experience changes in the composition of their outer membranes. These changes can include the disappearance of some of the "receptor" molecules that should be there to receive the chemical messages being sent by the cells' coworkers – preventing the cells from working together.

Is Brain Aging Inevitable?

Everyone seems to experience his or her own individual rate of decline in brain function. It is rapid in some and moderate in most, but barely noticeable in the "lucky" few. This observation begs the questions – what do they have and how can you get it? And just as important – if decline already has started, can it be turned around? What does the scientific evidence have to say?

Brain Aging is Not Inevitable

Declining cognitive performance is nearly universal after 70 years of age. However, any initial deficits do not mean that total loss is just around the corner. For example, in one study of elderly individuals with mild degrees of cognitive impairment at the beginning of the study, after 2 to 3 years only 20% had gotten worse while another 20% actually improved on their own – and the other 60% remained about the same.[1] Other reports[2-5] confirm the conclusion that initially mild cognitive decline can stabilize or even be reversed. While we will get into this discussion later, maintaining a healthy antioxidant to pro-oxidant balance may be an important factor in maintaining cognitive health with age. This includes wise lifestyle choices, ensuring antioxidant-rich dietary intake and smart supplementation with nutrients that support brain health.

Essential Brain Nourishment

Energy, Vitamins and Minerals

Your brain needs energy – and lots of it! This small part of your body accounts for about 20% or more of your total energy use every day and is the major reason your liver works so hard to make other compounds into **glucose**, your brain's major fuel. Proper brain function requires ample amounts of glucose to be readily-available within the brain. Concentration, focusing, attention, short-term memory, long-term memory, recall and reaction time are all essential brain activities and require ample amounts of energy. Not only must there be enough

> *"Maintaining a healthy antioxidant to pro-oxidant balance may be an important factor in maintaining cognitive health with age."*

glucose in the brain, it must be able to convert that glucose into metabolic energy extremely rapidly and efficiently. That process requires several cofactors, including the B-vitamins and several minerals – thiamin, biotin, riboflavin, pantothenic acid, niacin, magnesium, zinc, iron and calcium. Too little of any *one* of these nutrients in the brain and glucose metabolism can slow, leading to impaired brain functions.[6] In addition, the structural integrity of the neuronal network that allows the level of electrical and chemical activity that occurs in a healthy brain to proceed without mishap requires abundant supplies of riboflavin, vitamin B_{12}, vitamin B_6, folic acid, pantothenic acid, iron and zinc. Recently published research shows that combining B-vitamins with N-acetylcysteine dramatically improved the cognitive abilities of a series of elderly men and women.[7]

Fish Oils

The fish oil, docosahexaenoic acid (DHA), is the major polyunsaturated fatty acid in the brain. Between 25% and 50% of all the fatty acids in the brain, optic nerve and retina are DHA. One of the functions of DHA in the brain is to stimulate brain neurons to maintain strong cell-to-cell contacts so that they may communicate with ease. When DHA is added to the diet it enters the brain and is incorporated into those areas of neuron cell membranes where cells are in proximity and exchange messages. When the neuronal membrane DHA content is increased in rats, they learn more quickly and exhibit increased curiosity about their environment – all signs of enhanced cognitive functions. In elderly men and women, the ability to retain cognitive functions may increase as daily fish oil intake increases.[8] DHA and other essential fatty acids support several structural components of brain tissue.

> *"Between 25% and 50% of all the fatty acids in the brain, optic nerve and retina are DHA."*

Phosphatidylserine

While DHA is the major fatty acid in the brain, phosphatidylserine is the major structural component of brain cell membranes. Phosphatidylserine also is a precursor to phosphatidylcholine, another structural component of cell membranes. Within the neuronal cell membrane, phosphatidylserine is required in order for the chemical events through which one neuron communicates with another to occur. Enhancing the concentration of phosphatidylserine in neurons increases the speed and accuracy of cell-to-cell communication – effects that manifest as enhanced performance on tasks that test learning ability and short-term memory. Phosphatidylserine facilitates the formation of new memories (learning) and their retrieval.

In a "gold standard" randomized placebo-controlled clinical trial, daily dietary supplementation with 300 mg of phosphatidylserine has been found to produce significant improvements in attention, vigilance, short-term recall, immediate memory, vocabulary skills and the ability to recall words in men and women over 60 years of age.[9] In other studies, moderate losses of the abilities to concentrate, focus attention, learn and perform daily activities were somewhat reversed by daily supplementation with 300 mg of phosphatidylserine; in particular, verbal recall, long-term memory and overall cognitive functioning were improved.[10,11]

Daily dietary supplementation with 100 mg to 300 mg of phosphatidylserine enhances human cognitive function and may interrupt, attenuate or arrest cognitive deterioration. This property of phosphatidylserine was recognized by the U.S. Food and Drug Administration in its announcement of a Qualified Health Claim on May 13, 2003, that "Consumption of phosphatidylserine may reduce the risk of dementia in the elderly" and "Consumption of phosphatidylserine may reduce the risk of cognitive dysfunction in the elderly."[12] In making its determination, the U.S. Food and Drug Administration also endorsed the safety of daily dietary supplementation with up to 300 mg of phosphatidylserine.[12]

Ginkgo biloba Leaf Extract

Extracts of the leaves of Ginkgo biloba, the world's oldest living tree, contain a range of phytonutrients that stimulate the cholinergic neurotransmitter system. In one randomized, double-blind, placebo-controlled study, 30 days of daily dietary supplementation with the extract produced improvements in the speed of information processing by working memory and the accuracy of executive processing in young men and women who were otherwise completely normal in their cognitive abilities.[13] In an older study, the one-time consumption of 600 mg of *Ginkgo biloba* leaf extract increased memory performance in healthy young women with "good" memories within one hour.[14] More recent research showed that acute administration of a single dose of *Ginkgo biloba* to young, healthy individuals led to significant performance enhancements for sustained-attention tasks and pattern recognition tasks 4 hours after dosing.[15] Furthermore, a study performed in elderly individuals consuming 120 mg of a Gingko biloba extract daily for one year found that the extract was able to aid in the maintenance of cognitive function over the study period.[16] The extract was extremely safe and in several cases was shown to enhance cognitive ability in the study group. The results of these studies illustrate the promotion of mental functioning by *Ginkgo biloba* leaf extract.

Choline

Choline is a B-vitamin-like nutrient that is required for the synthesis of essential components of nerve and brain cell membranes. In humans, the rate of synthesis of these components is governed by the availability of choline in the brain, which itself is determined by dietary choline intake. When incoming supplies of choline are inadequate, existing neuronal cell membranes will be "cannibalized" for their choline – obviously a losing proposition in the long run. In contrast, dietary supplementation with choline prevents such avoidable loss of brain cell integrity. The current Recommended Dietary Allowances for choline range from 125 mg/day for neonatal infants to 425 mg/day for adults and 550 mg/day for lactating women. Daily intakes of up to 3500 mg are safe.[17]

Glycerophosphocholine (GPC)

Within neurons in the brain, phosphatidylcholine is a vital membrane phospholipid that participates in ensuring effective interneuronal communication. When brain cells interact they sometimes form new connections by "reaching out" to their neighbors with an extension of themselves – a section of new cellular material that must be wrapped properly in membrane material. At other times, peroxidation of a portion of neuronal membrane requires its removal and replacement. Both new construction and remodeling require a plentiful supply of new phosphatidylcholine. Some of this building material is made fresh from nutrients supplied by the blood, but most is produced by recycling the phosphatidylcholine obtained from the existing membrane material.

GPC Supplies Choline to the Brain

The first step in the recycling process is to break down phosphatidylcholine into its individual components, one of which is L- -glycerophosphocholine (GPC).[18] As research published in the *Journal of Biological Chemistry* has shown, the choline from GPC can be recovered by the cell and reused to produce fresh phosphatidylcholine where it is needed.[19] In addition, the choline that is released from GPC within the neuron can be used to produce acetylcholine, the neurotransmitter chemical without which much of your brain activity would be impossible.

GPC Works with Choline

If for some reason not enough choline is available to support the need for new acetylcholine, brain cells will "cannibalize" their own membranes, tearing out phosphatidylcholine to get at its choline. The results of a study published recently in *Mechanisms of Ageing and Development* show that, within brain cells, supplemental GPC is a better source of choline than is dietary choline.[20] Adequate GPC availability prevents neuronal self-destruction from occurring.

GPC Promotes Mental Processing

The results of several studies indicate that GPC promotes effective mental performance. For example, GPC has enhanced the balance between the various types of brain waves, has decreased reaction time (reflecting faster mental reactions) and has supported cell-to-cell communication within the brain of middle-aged men and women. These physiological effects have been expressed as improvements in mental functioning abilities in elderly men and women consuming 1200 mg of GPC daily.[21] The author of an extensive analysis of published randomized placebo-controlled human clinical trials published in *Mechanisms of Ageing and Development* concluded that daily dietary supplementation with 1200 mg of GPC promotes healthy memory and attention processes in the human brain and supports emotional stability.[22]

Neuroprotection

Neuroprotection is a term that describes mechanisms to protect the brain from oxidative damage.[23] The brain is an organ that is especially sensitive to oxidative stress, and many of the biochemical and metabolic changes that accumulate with advancing age act to increase the oxidative stress on the human brain. Increased oxidative stress has a harmful impact on cognitive functioning and, as discussed above, is a major cause of brain aging.

> *"Increased oxidative stress has a harmful impact on cognitive functioning and is a major cause of brain aging."*

The need for additional neuroprotection will accompany any situation in which brain metabolism is increased – such as during learning, thinking or any of the other cognitive processes. There is evidence suggesting that inadequate neuroprotection is part of the set of factors that can impair learning, memory, attention and concentration. On the other hand, increasing neuroprotective capacity may be able to prevent these impairments and could even foster the repair of oxidative damage in the brain.

Vinpocetine

Vinpocetine is a substance that protects neurons from oxidative damage. In addition, vinpocetine acts as a cerebral vasodilator that enhances circulation to the brain. Increased oxygen and nutrient supply to the brain can enhance cognitive functioning ability; in several experiments, 10 mg of vinpocetine has increased the ability to distinguish discrete sensory data, reduced reaction time and enhanced short-term memory functions (retention and recall).[24,25] Furthermore, vinpocetine has been found to have free radical scavenging effects at concentrations that are achievable in humans, with dose-dependant antioxidant activity capable of protecting the integrity of brain tissues.[26] The dual action of vinpocetine to enhance brain oxygenation and support antioxidant protection of brain structures makes vinpocetine a unique nutrient for cognitive support.

Acetyl-L-Carnitine

Acetyl-L-carnitine is a modified version of L-carnitine that is transported into the brain where it acts as a strong antioxidant. This property was demonstrated in research published recently in Neuropharmacology.[27] In that experiment, nerve cells became more resistant to oxidative attack when acetyl-L-carnitine was available to them.

The neuroprotective properties of acetyl-L-carnitine are associated with beneficial effects on cognitive functioning. As shown in a "gold standard" randomized placebo-controlled clinical trial, elderly men and women with very mild age-related cognitive decline who supplemented their diets with 2000 mg of acetyl-L-carnitine enjoyed significant improvements in short-term memory, long-term memory, attention span and verbal fluency.[28,29] A meta-analysis including 21 clinical trails using acetyl-L-carnitine was published in 2003. The results showed that the nutrient had significant positive benefits when compared to placebo treatment for supporting cognitive ability in humans.[30]

Vitamin E

Because it acts within cell membranes, vitamin E has the potential to play a major neuroprotective role in the human brain. Scientists have reported that the ability of elderly men and women to perform on tests of cognitive functioning was greatest in those with the highest daily consumption of vitamin E.[31] The recently-published results of a detailed analysis of published studies show that daily dietary supplementation with 200 IU to 400 IU of vitamin E reduce the risk of certain neurological concerns characterized by oxidation of neuronal membrane lipids.[32] Given its antioxidant prowess, vitamin E plays an essential role in supporting brain function.

> *"Scientists have reported that the ability of elderly men and women to perform on tests of cognitive functioning was greatest in those with the highest daily consumption of vitamin E."*

Selenium

The water-soluble counterpart to vitamin E, selenium is a required activating agent for a set of antioxidant enzymes that contribute to the neuroprotection of the human brain.[33] The activity of these powerful quenchers of free electrons depends on the amount of selenium that is available as a cofactor through the diet and through dietary supplements.

Brain Inflammation

The human brain seems to develop a state of chronic low-grade inflammation after a number of decades of life.[34] The ravages of free radical accumulation become detectable with increasing age. In this state, the chemical messages being exchanged by the activated immune system of the brain have the side-effect of occasionally interfering with neuronal function.[35] Therefore, the dietary agents that help modulate free radical production, contained within fruits and vegetables, and fish, in particular, may be useful in helping your brain ward off some of the influences that could be contributing to its accelerated aging. Adding several brain health boosters to your daily regimen, in the form of dietary supplements, can provide further support in your quest to protect the fundamental functions of the brain throughout life.

Brain Health Boosters

- B-Vitamins
- Magnesium
- Zinc
- Iron
- N-Acetylcysteine
- Fish Oils
- Phosphatidylserine
- *Ginkgo biloba* leaf extract
- Glycerophosphocholine (GPC)
- Choline
- Vinpocetine
- Acetyl-L-Carnitine
- Vitamin E
- Selenium
- Vitamin C
- Quercetin
- Resveratrol
- Pomegranate Juice
- Carotenoids
- Pycnogenol®
- Fruits and Vegetables

20

Blood Sugar – Healthy Support for Optimal Levels

As the development and progression of unhealthy blood glucose metabolism can often take years, it is important to establish and inculcate practices early on which can support healthy blood sugar metabolism.

Powerful Practices to Promote a Healthy Relationship between You and Sugar

You can take charge of your body's struggle to control glucose. Implementing these powerful practices can promote healthy blood sugar metabolism as a part of your diet.

Eat Less Sugar and Eat It More Slowly

The "sugar load" you place on your body directly reflects how much sugar and starch you eat – the more glucose in any form that you eat or drink, digest, absorb and send into your blood, the more you need to work to get the glucose into your cells. Thus, eating less simple carbohydrates and processed foods, while eating more complex carbohydrates and fiber-rich foods, can lead to decreased absorption of sugar from meals and better overall blood sugar regulation. Why make your blood sugar-regulation system work any harder than is necessary?

Establish and Maintain a Healthy Body Weight

As is confirmed by recently published research body fat interferes with insulin's ability to stimulate your muscle cells to remove glucose from your blood.[1] The more fat you're carrying, the less able you are to maintain healthy blood glucose regulation. Period. No more discussion. No excuses. Maintaining a healthy body weight through diet and exercise facilitates proper sugar utilization. Get your weight right and help keep your blood glucose under control. It's that simple.

DASH to Glucose Health

Lifestyle changes that incorporate a combination of weight loss, reduced sodium intake, increased physical activity, moderation of alcohol intake and a diet high in fruits, vegetables and low-fat dairy products (low in total fat, saturated fat, and cholesterol contents; high in magnesium, calcium and protein contents) – the "DASH" Lifestyle – dramatically improve insulin sensitivity in older adults who are not yet hyperglycemic. Even simply increasing the number of servings of fruits and vegetables consumed daily to 5 (still below the recommended 7 to 9 servings) has been shown to provide powerful protection to the blood glucose regulatory system. So has cutting back to only one serving of red meat daily. Of course, so has consuming the recommended amount of dietary fiber which, according to a recent study, can improve insulin sensitivity by about 10% and contribute to sustained maintenance of healthy blood glucose control into the future.[2] The merits of this lifestyle approach have

> *"The more fat you're carrying, the less able you are to maintain healthy blood glucose regulation."*

been reinforced by the findings in a study published recently in the *American Journal of Clinical Nutrition* – limiting yourself to only one serving of French fries a week significantly enhances chances of having healthy blood glucose control.[3]

Add the Correct Mix of Minerals –

The US Food and Drug Administration approved a Qualified Health Claim for chromium – they agreed that daily dietary supplementation with chromium picolinate (with more than 50 mcg of chromium) can improve insulin sensitivity and restore and maintain healthy blood glucose regulation and homeostasis.[4] The US Food and Drug Administration also has determined that daily chromium picolinate may reduce the risk of developing adult onset ("type 2") diabetes later in life.[4] The results of a human clinical trial published recently in *Fertility and Sterility* confirm that dietary supplementation with chromium picolinate (1000 mcg of chromium daily) dramatically supports the maintenance of healthy blood glucose regulation and protects it from destabilizing influences.[5]

Adequate intake of the important mineral magnesium is required for maintenance of stable insulin sensitivity. In individuals with normal fasting blood glucose and insulin concentrations, fasting plasma insulin concentration goes down as dietary magnesium intake goes up – a principle that was confirmed again in the results of a study published recently in *Diabetes Care.*[6] In other words, as magnesium intake increases, less insulin is needed to help muscle cells obtain glucose from the blood. The longer you can maintain a high degree of insulin efficiency, the longer you maintain adequate blood glucose regulation capacity. As shown in a 6-year study of 39,345 women, a 12-year study of 42,872 men and an 18-year study of 85,060 women – adults who routinely consume at least 300 mg of magnesium daily have healthier glucose metabolism over the years and are more likely to maintain health with age.

The little-known trace mineral, vanadium, also plays important roles in promoting healthy blood sugar control. Vanadium may also protect other tissues against the potential consequences of chronically dysregulated blood sugar. In a study of rat eyes published recently in the *Journal of Biosciences*, vanadium protected the lens from the destructive effects of overexposure to glucose.[7] In live rats, vanadium supplementation has prevented disruptions in glucose regulation caused by a diabetes-inducing drug. While these studies were in diseased animals, vanadium may also be of utility in healthy humans. As an example, supplementation with 150 mg of vanadium (as vanadyl sulfate) daily has been shown to increase the ability to move glucose from the blood into muscle cells – promoting the sustained normalization of blood glucose regulation in human subjects.

It seems that minerals function in synergy with one another – vanadium contributes to blood glucose regulation by facilitating the regulatory actions of magnesium, while magnesium enables chromium to increase the insulin sensitivity of muscle cells.

A Note of Caution – Never become confused by thinking that dietary ingredients such as chromium, magnesium or vanadium, effective components of a comprehensive healthy blood glucose maintenance program, can substitute for hypoglycemic drugs if your blood glucose already is out of control. As shown by the results of a human clinical trial published recently in *Diabetes Care*, maintaining healthy blood glucose regulation is not the same as restoring regulation by the treatment of an existing disease.[8] Thus, take your minerals to help keep you healthy before your sugar levels are to the point where they may not do much good.

Sprinkle on the Cinnamon

Cinnamon can facilitate the normal action of insulin. In men and women, 1 to 6 g of cinnamon daily maintained normal blood sugar levels in a study that reinforced the expectation that cinnamon consumption can contribute to the maintenance of healthy blood sugar regulation and insulin sensitivity. However, the results of a human clinical trial published recently in the *Journal of Nutrition* suggest that small amounts of cinnamon (less than 3 g daily) may not contribute to the maintenance of healthy sugar metabolism.[9] It appears that the benefits of cinnamon adhere to the time-honored culinary principle that too little spice is without effect. However, a small study conducted using a particular water-soluble cinnamon extract showed significant benefits on blood sugar levels and body composition. The results of the study pointed out that individuals supplemented with 500 mg per day of the extract had healthier fasting blood sugar levels and a statistically significant decrease in body fat than individuals in the placebo group when the extract was given as a part of a healthy diet.[10]

Dark Chocolate in Moderation

How can something that tastes so good be so healthy? According to the results of a study published recently in the *American Journal of Clinical Nutrition*, faithful daily consumption of 4 ounces of dark chocolate (containing about 500 mg of quercetin and mixed catechins) helped maintain normal sensitivity to insulin, contributing to healthy blood sugar control.[11] One caution – this much dark chocolate will add about 500 calories to your daily caloric intake. Remember to adjust your dietary intake of calories – and exercise more – instead of just adding the chocolate!

Herbal Support for Healthy Blood Sugar

Extracts of the leaves of the herb *Gymnema sylvestre* contain phytonutrients that promote and sustain healthy blood sugar concentrations. Gymnema is an herb that has been used traditionally in the Ayurvedic herbal system to support normal blood sugar levels and has been researched in animals and humans.[12] This herb acts in part by slowing the rate of absorption of the sugar in foods and beverages. However, because this herbal extract also may act in part by stimulating some insulin secretion by the pancreas and by itself could contribute to hyperinsulinemia, it should not be consumed alone but only in combination with the other dietary ingredients that increase the efficiency of insulin action in muscle and stimulate glucose entry into muscle cells.

Fenugreek seeds contain 4-hydroxyisoleucine, an amino acid-like phytonutrient that increases muscle cell sensitivity to insulin and facilitates the maintenance of long-term glucose homeostasis. Findings published recently in *Molecular and Cellular Biochemistry* confirmed the results of a number of previous studies by showing that Fenugreek seed powder promotes sustained normalization of blood glucose regulation.[13] Similarly, the daily consumption of several grams of powdered Fenugreek seeds has been found to contribute to the stabilization and maintenance of healthy fasting plasma glucose concentrations and oral glucose tolerance (ability to move glucose from the blood into muscle cells) in men and women. In addition, a study of rat eyes published recently in *Molecular and Cellular Biochemistry* found that Fenugreek seed powder protected the lens and retina from the destructive effects of overexposure to glucose.[14] These reports demonstrate that Fenugreek seed powder promotes 1) normalization of blood glucose regulation, 2) protective glucose homeostasis in the tissues most susceptible to permanent hyperglycemic damage and 3) stabilization and maintenance of healthy oral glucose tolerance. Thus adding herbs like *Gymnema sylvestre* as a dietary supplement, and incorporating spices like Fenugreek and others to your diet, can lead to long-term healthy regulation of blood sugar metabolism.

Phytonutrients for Healthy Blood Sugar Maintenance

The findings of two recently published studies indicate that the phytonutrients (*not* the caffeine) in both regular and "decaf" coffees are beneficial in the maintenance of healthy blood glucose regulation.[15,16] In fact, the more coffee these 117,071 American women drank on a regular basis, day in, day out, year after year, the better their regulation of blood glucose metabolism. Coffee contains chlorogenic acid and trigonelline, its two major phytonutrient components. A recent study found that acute intake of chlorogenic acid and trigonelline in 15 men was found to significantly reduce blood sugar levels as assessed by performance of an oral glucose tolerance test (OGTT) compared to placebo.[17]

> *"Maintaining blood sugar levels in an ideal range is an important cornerstone for health and wellness."*

Maintaining blood sugar levels in an ideal range is an important cornerstone for health and wellness. Healthy blood sugar regulation can be achieved by implementing several dietary measures, incorporating exercise and other healthy lifestyle practices into your daily routine, and by adding health-promoting nutritional supplements to your daily regimen.

21

Healthy Circulation: Go with the Flow

Healthy blood circulation through the cardiovascular system depends on two major factors. The first factor that needs to be in place is a healthy heart. The heart is the pump that keeps blood moving throughout the body. The second major factor that's necessary is healthy arteries and veins. The blood vessels serve as the conduits for blood to flow to the tissues. Akin to a highway network, the veins and arteries that make up the passageways of the circulatory system need to be made up of healthy cells and need to be clean and unclogged with traffic. There are a number of issues that can affect healthy circulation. Let's look at a few of the major ones.

Blood Sugar Control and Circulation

High blood sugar (hyperglycemia) allows too much sugar to interact with the proteins that line the inner walls of your blood vessels. In your blood vessels, sugar + protein = AGE (advanced glycation endproducts – sugar-protein complexes that destroy the function of the protein and act as "debris" stuck to the blood vessel walls – sort of like rust along the inside of a pipe). This traffic can block flow and prevent capillaries from nourishing our cells. Several ways to ensure blood sugar levels stay healthy include dietary measures such as a low-sugar low-starch diet with plenty of fruits and vegetables, maintaining a healthy body weight, and dietary supplementation with nutrients like chromium, magnesium, vanadium and extracts of *Gymnema sylvestre* and Fenugreek.

Maintain Arterial Health

Blood can't get to those healthy capillaries if it can't get through your arteries. Keep them wide open by adopting sensible dietary measures such as cutting back on red meats and animal fats. Instead, increase consumption of fatty cold-water fish and fresh garlic cloves (or plenty of garlic powder) plus abundant amounts of fruits and vegetables every day. In addition, daily dietary supplementation with high-quality fish oils, allicin (from garlic), vitamin C, vitamin E, *N*-acetylcysteine, quercetin, resveratrol and phytonutrients from pomegranates supports arterial health and structure.

Sipping a cup or two of vessel health-promoting green tea is also beneficial, as green tea is a rich source of antioxidants and polyphenols that promote blood vessel health.

"Just as important as getting fresh nutritious blood out to your cells is getting the nutrient-depleted blood back to your heart for another cycle."

Support Venous Flow

Just as important as getting fresh nutritious blood out to your cells is getting the nutrient-depleted blood back to your heart for another cycle. Keep your venous return systems flowing smoothly with daily dietary supplementation of nutrients such as diosmin, hesperidin, Pycnogenol®, resveratrol, and horse chestnut seed extract.

Horse Chestnut Seed extract

Often, cells in the walls of the veins become "loose" and leaky with age, allowing for fluids to leak out into the surrounding tissue. While it probably happens inside tissues where its effects cannot be seen, weakness in the veins is most visible when it occurs under or in the skin.

Horse chestnut extract has been recognized for many years as a "tonic for the veins." Modern research has discovered that horse chestnut extract indeed "tightens up" the spaces between cells in the walls of veins, decreasing leakage. A recently published study showed that horse chestnut extract stimulates mild lateral contraction within the walls of veins, effectively "sealing up" any gaps that might have formed.[1]

Scientists also reported in the *Journal of Veterinary Medical Science* that horse chestnut extract contains inhibitors of enzymes that may cause vein health to be compromised when activated.[2] Its inhibition of these important enzymes may explain the ability of horse chestnut extract to enhance venous structure and flow.

The prestigious Cochrane Collaboration has performed 2 intensive analyses of horse chestnut extract (most recently in 2006) and both times has concluded that horse chestnut extract is "efficacious and safe" in promoting healthy veins.[3]

The experts agree – horse chestnut extract helps to seal leaky veins and is a valuable contributor to every effort to keep your veins and circulatory system healthy.

Diosmin and Hesperidin

Research in Europe has identified a flavonoid compound that supports vein health by providing the benefits that aging blood vessels crave. The phytonutrient diosmin is found in several plants and also can be made from hesperidin, a flavonoid found in the skins of citrus fruits. In commercial products these two flavonoids are combined in a 9:1 ratio of 450 mg of diosmin and 50 mg of hesperidin. When tested in men and women needing nutritional venous support because of age, dietary supplementation with

450 mg of diosmin and 50 mg of hesperidin twice a day for 2 to 6 months improved measures of venous flow and allowed for superior maintenance of healthy vein structure.[4]

The results of an analysis of published research describing the effects of diosmin plus hesperidin used in combination for venous support were published recently in *Angiology*.[5] The analysis showed that dietary supplementation with 450 mg of diosmin and 50 mg of hesperidin twice a day for 6 months produced venous healing and powerfully supported the beneficial effects of diosmin and hesperidin on blood vessels.

A "gold standard" randomized double-blind placebo controlled human clinical trial demonstrated that diosmin alone (450 mg twice a day for 60 days) has strong benefits for leg veins and comfort that older adults generally experience due to decreased venous function.[4]

Hesperidin is additionally revered as a strong tissue-supporting antioxidant. Free radical damage to veins leads to many of the vein-related health issues seen today in clinical practice. Adding hesperidin to diosmin thus creates a combination that potently supports venous health by providing protection against free radical attack.

Support of Blood Vessels throughout the Body

In addition to veins in the legs needing nutritional support, blood vessels of other areas of the body require adequate nutrition to function optimally. This includes the veins of the rectum and anus, which require extra flexibility and strength in order to be able to withstand and adapt to the large fluctuations in pressures they experience during normal bowel movements. If their walls become weakened due to lack of nutrition, they can collapse and stretch. Obviously, antioxidant support for these overworked blood vessels should be expected to help them maintain structural integrity and avoid failure. Fortunately, dietary supplementation with 450 mg of diosmin and 50 mg of hesperidin twice a day has been shown to dramatically support the blood vessels of these areas as well.

One More Thing –

Help your heart in its strenuous work by doing some standing and stretching exercises several times a day, drinking copious amounts of water, and avoiding constrictive clothes, salty foods and excessive alcoholic beverages. A regular routine of cardiovascular exercise would also go a long way in providing added support to the entire cardiovascular system.

Diosmin, Hesperidin & Horse Chestnut

- Diosmin has been shown in research studies to support venous tone and normal lymphatic drainage.*
- Both Hesperidin and Diosmin may modulate the level and activity of certain immune factors, thus supporting the normal healthy function of blood vessels.*
- Diosmin (in the proper concentration) has been shown to promote efficient circulatory and vascular function.*
- A combination of Hesperidin and Diosmin has been shown in clinical studies to support healthy venous tone and normal vessel elasticity, thereby supporting healthy circulation.*
- Horse Chestnut Seed extract has been shown to exert significant antioxidant effects on vascular tissue, allowing for enhancement of normal circulatory function and the support of healthy vessel tone.*
- Studies point to the potential ability of horse chestnut seed extract to modulate the effects of enzymes in the circulatory system to promote normal, healthy vascular function.*

22

Eye Health - Seeing is Believing

Vision and eyesight often receive little attention when it comes to nutrition. The vast majority of people are unaware that there are foods and nutritional support ingredients that can promote healthy vision as they get older. Whether you prefer to add selected fruits and vegetables to your diet, supplement your diet with an appropriate high-quality formula, or both, the foundation of eye health is the combination of several ingredients that prevent free radical destruction of eye tissue over the long run to maintain healthy visual function with age. These include basic antioxidants such as vitamins C and E, -carotene, and the mineral zinc (balanced with copper); two vastly under-appreciated phytonutrients – lutein and zeaxanthin; the extract of French maritime pine bark – Pycnogenol® – and potentially the structural-support nutrient hyaluronic acid. These powerful nutritional support champions form the basis of every healthy vision regimen.

Antioxidants -Carotene, vitamins C, E and Zinc

The AREDS (Age-Related Eye Disease Study) trial was conducted several years ago under the sponsorship of the National Eye Institute, which is a part of the National Institutes of Health. The trial was conducted to evaluate the effect of supplementation with antioxidant vitamins and the mineral zinc in supporting eye health in aging individuals. The AREDS study involved 4,757 participants aged between 55 and 80 years old. The results of the study were released in October 2001. The study participants supplemented with either antioxidants alone, zinc alone, or the combination of antioxidants plus zinc for an average of 6.3 years. The group supplementing with the combination had the best outcomes with statistically significant results in maintaining normal visual acuity over that period of time.[1]

The formula used in the study included 500 mg of vitamin C, 400 IU of vitamin E, 15 mg of -carotene, 80 mg of zinc and 2 mg of copper supplemented on a daily basis. This study was integral in showing that a relatively high dose of antioxidant nutrients was able to help promote healthy vision in elderly individuals, and suggests the benefits of antioxidant supplementation to eye health.

The human retina contains the photoreceptor cells that convert light into vision. A healthy retina is absolutely vital to good vision. Oxidative damage to the eye is the most common cause of vision problems and loss in adulthood.[2] Preventing oxidative damage before it happens is the best protection you can give your eyes.

Lutein, Zeaxanthin and the Retina

Fortunately, the retina contains lutein and zeaxanthin, the carotenoid cousins of β-carotene. Lutein and zeaxanthin absorb ultraviolet light – a powerful antioxidant effect that protects the retina from oxidative damage. The absorption of ultraviolet light before it reaches the photoreceptors also helps to keep the visual image clear and distortion-free. By absorbing ultraviolet light, lutein and zeaxanthin contribute to visual acuity.

"Oxidative damage to the eye is the most common cause of vision problems and loss in adulthood."

Smoke in Your Eyes (a bad thing)

Smoking has detrimental effects all around. Several tissues can suffer oxidative damage as a result of exposure to several of the compounds present in cigarette smoke. Direct exposure to cigarette smoke causes oxidation in the eye and its internal structures, and can double the retina's need for the carotenoids lutein and zeaxanthin.

Age-Related Changes in Vision

Age also increases the retinal requirement for lutein and zeaxanthin, which approximately doubles between the ages of 20 and 80 years.[3] Elderly men and women with low amounts of retinal lutein and zeaxanthin experience a decline in visual acuity and are much more likely to suffer age-related visual stress. Daily dietary supplementation with as little as 6 mg of lutein is a powerful promoter of visual acuity and eye health.[4,5]

Of course, "age-related" refers less to the fact that an individual is getting older and more to the fact that there is oxidative damage to eye tissue, which can occur at any age and in any individual. Thus, ensuring adequate lutein intake can be beneficial for everyone.

Lutein, Zeaxanthin and the Lens

Oxidative damage to the structure of the eye known as the lens is also common. Lutein and zeaxanthin filter high-energy blue light and function as antioxidants in the lens – functions which can protect this essential eye structure from being damaged. Researchers found that women aged 53 to 73 years with daily lutein plus zeaxanthin intakes of at least 2.4 mg nearly doubled their chances of having optimally-functioning lenses.[6] Yet another reason for supplementing with these beneficial carotenoids.

Lutein, Zeaxanthin and the Optic Nerve

Making sure that your eyes contain enough of the natural antioxidants, lutein and zeaxanthin, can ensure continued support for optic nerve health. The optic nerve transmits visual information from retinal tissue to the brain. Thus, damage to the optic nerve can severely affect visual acuity. Ensuring adequate lutein and zeaxanthin intake can protect the optic nerve from free radical damage.

> *"Ensuring adequate lutein and zeaxanthin intake can protect the optic nerve from free radical damage."*

Lutein and Zeaxanthin – Where Do They Come From?

The lutein and zeaxanthin of the macular pigment are entirely of dietary origin (and therefore lutein and zeaxanthin are essential nutrients).[2] Lutein and zeaxanthin are found naturally in corn, broccoli, green beans, green peas, brussels sprouts, cabbage, kale, collard greens, spinach, lettuce, kiwi, honey dew, nettles, algae, the petals of many yellow flowers, the yolks of eggs laid by hens fed marigolds and high-quality dietary supplements. The results of a study published recently in the *Journal of Nutrition* indicate that more of the lutein (and probably zeaxanthin) that you consume can be absorbed if you add a little avocado.[7]

Recent studies have also confirmed that the more lutein and zeaxanthin one consumes, the more it can benefit eye health. Studies suggest that dietary intake of both carotenoids causes an increase in the amount of carotenoids reaching the eyes and thus able to confer protection from free radical damage.[8,9]

Pycnogenol®

As we know, the normal processes of vision and daily environmental exposures to eye tissue produce vast amounts of free radicals. Overload your eyes with these destructive byproducts of sight and you risk permanent damage to the retina, cornea and lens. Pycnogenol® protects the structures of the eye – the cornea, lens and retina – from vision-destroying oxidation.[10]

Incorporating eye-friendly nutrients into your daily nutritional regimen increases your chances of enjoying worry-free visual function throughout life. Antioxidant nutrients such as -carotene, vitamins C and E, Zinc, the carotenoids lutein and zeaxanthin, Pycnogenol® and hyaluronic acid can all play a part in ensuring you maintain healthy visual acuity and eye function by providing your visual organs with the nourishment and protection they desire.

23

Skin Health - Nourishing your Insides to Nourish your Outsides

Skin health is a direct reflection of health overall. What's on the inside is expressed on the outside. In many traditions worldwide, skin health has been related to "impurities" and "toxins" in the blood. Furthermore, several traditional medical systems advocate supporting the efficiency of the liver and detoxifying organs of the body as a means of enhancing skin health. It makes sense that an excessive level of "toxins" in circulation could potentially cause blemishes on the skin. Thus, supporting liver health as a means of supporting healthy skin is a viable approach.

Besides the liver, poor skin health has been related to digestive function. Our digestive tracts are one of the means for the outside world to make direct contact with our insides, especially in the realm of foods and diet. It's also where many of our food intolerances are developed, either because of immune deficiencies or because of defects in our digestive capacities. Another contributing factor is bacteria and yeast that normally populate our digestive tract. If the bacterial flora is health-promoting, they help digest our food and aid in extracting skin-healthy nutrients from the diet. If the bacterial flora is unhealthy, we fail to take full advantage of the nutrients contained within the foods we eat. Unhealthy bacteria and yeast can also excrete toxins into the gut that can add to the toxic burden our bodies have to deal with, eventually affecting the health of our skin.

A further aspect related to skin health that is important to keep in mind is that the skin itself is a major barrier, which shields and protects our bodies from the ravages of our environment. Intact skin functions to protect us from potential insults that we are exposed to in the world in which we live. Damaged skin compromises this protective shield, leading to compromises in immune defenses and other health problems.

> "Unhealthy bacteria and yeast can also excrete toxins into the gut that can add to the toxic burden our bodies have to deal with, eventually affecting the health of our skin."

When considering supporting skin health, think about nourishing the skin (and body) from within. What's healthy for the body is healthy for the skin. Ensuring that our diets contain nutrients that are healthy and support the structural needs of the skin is the first step. The next step is to ensure optimal digestive function and to ramp up the detoxifying ability of the liver. Finally, limiting the effects of environmental exposures that can compromise skin health is also important.

Keeping Healthy Skin Healthy

Healthy skin is smooth, soft, and supple, with a nice uniform color and the sheen of youthfulness. Discolorations and other blemishes aren't just unsightly – they alert you to the less-than-optimal health status of your natural outer covering. The beneficial effects of your favorite creams, which contribute important nutrients and hydration from the outside, can be augmented by including several skin-friendly nutrients in your diet.

Pycnogenol® to Enhance Venous Tone and Circulation

Pycnogenol® strengthens the ability of small blood vessels in the skin to resist oxidative damage.[1] Results of recently published human clinical trials confirm the power of Pycnogenol® to promote healthy, well-nourished skin by supporting healthy circulation and vein health.[2,3] Pycnogenol® also contains compounds that have potent antioxidant properties to support the skin's immune defenses.

Hyaluronic Acid for Skin Elasticity

Aging skin contains less hyaluronic acid. Because hyaluronic acid is the most abundant water-binding glycosaminoglycan in healthy skin, loss of hyaluronic acid results in loss of elasticity and increased density – giving skin a dry and wrinkled appearance. Adding hyaluronic acid back to skin increases its moisture content and flexibility.

Exposure to sunlight also dries skin and reduces its flexibility. Increasing the hyaluronic acid content of skin increases its resistance to the deleterious effects of sunlight. A paper published recently in the *Journal of Pharmacology and Pharmaceutical Science* has shown hyaluronic acid to be a powerful antioxidant within the skin that prevents wrinkle-producing free radical damage of the skin as well as maintaining the normal level of hydration within the skin.[4]

"...pomegranate extract blocks the effects of ultraviolet light on the chemical pathways in the skin that can produce the unsightly signs of skin aging."

Hyaluronic acid promotes flexible and supple skin, which makes it an ideal candidate for your skin anti-aging program.

Smooth Out Your Coloration with Nutrition

Extracts of pomegranate fruit can help decrease your skin's tendency to develop spotty pigmentation after exposure to sunlight. In research published recently in *Bioscience, Biotechnology and Biochemistry*, the consumption of pomegranate extract prevented much of the excess pigmentation that otherwise was caused by sunlight exposure.[5] Other research published recently in *Photochemistry and Photobiology* has shown that pomegranate extract blocks the effects of ultraviolet light on the chemical pathways in the skin that can produce the unsightly signs of skin aging.[6]

Discolored spots on the skin can be caused by excessive oxidation within the skin – usually triggered by unprotected exposure to a little too much sun. Those great antioxidant vitamins, vitamin C and vitamin E, can intercept runaway melanin production in your skin – a major cause of the undesirable appearance of photoaged skin. But these vitamins never are as powerful as when they are combined with other targeted nutrients such as melatonin, which works in concert with the antioxidant vitamins to keep skin from overreacting to sunlight.

Another key to healthy skin is filling your diet with colorful phytonutrients! A growing body of research shows that men and women who supplement their diets with β-carotene, lutein and lycopene (along with vitamin C and vitamin E) can increase the ability of their skin to withstand sunlight without burning – powerful additional antioxidant support for a good sunscreen!

Stay Cool and Remain Refreshed – Both Are Good for Your Skin

Iced tea is for beating the heat inside your body – and it also helps you handle the sun's energy on the outside. Iced tea, and especially green tea, adds nutrients to your skin that increase its natural barrier to sunlight penetration. Research findings published recently in the *Chinese Medical Journal* and in the *Journal of Nutrition* testify to the protective properties of the phytonutrients in tea and especially in green tea.[7,8] It turns out green tea contains phytochemicals that have superb antioxidant activity. This property of tea allows it to confer potent protection to skin cells.

Lose Excess Fat for a Trimmer Appearance and More Supple Skin

You knew that if you could get yourself to limit your intake of fats you could drop a few pounds and trim your shape. You also need to know that that excess layer of fat you have built up between your skin and the rest of your body acts to dry out and stiffen your skin.[9] Take home message – don't take the fat home – leave it in the store or restaurant and help your skin draw admiration to your entire appearance.

Fish Oil for Skin Cell Communication

The essential fatty acids contained in fish oil are extremely beneficial for the skin. Our diets generally contain a large proportion of unhealthy fats and a high percentage of omega-6 fatty acids. However, cell membranes preferentially use the omega-3 fats from fish for incorporation into their membranes. These fats facilitate cell-to-cell communication and enhance the ability of cells to flush toxins out and push nutrients in, keeping cells healthy. While this is the case with cells throughout the body, this is also certainly true for skin cells. Thus, for truly vibrant skin, eat wild-caught fish that is loaded with omega-3 oils and supplement with a high-quality fish oil supplement.

Healthy Bacteria = Healthy Skin

Digestive function can have a big impact on skin health. Probiotic organisms are bacteria that produce beneficial health effects in the body and support optimal digestive function and nutrient absorption. Thus, supplementing with probiotics can have beneficial effects on the skin as they facilitate nutrient utilization by the body. See the Digestive Health chapter for more information on the health benefits of probiotics.

Support the Liver, Support the Skin

The liver is the major detoxifier of the body. Keeping the blood free and clear of toxins can have a large effect on the appearance of the skin. By enhancing the liver's detoxifying efficiency, you can ensure that toxins in circulation are properly neutralized. Herbs such as milk thistle and turmeric, and nutrients such as N-acetylcysteine and other antioxidants, play a role in supporting liver function. See the Liver Support chapter for more information on liver-healthy practices.

Supporting the skin begins with promoting the health of the digestive tract and liver, and providing optimal levels of nutrients that directly support skin health. Incorporating skin healthy dietary practices and therapeutic nutrients into your daily regimen can leave your skin supple, youthful, and glowing. The skin is a reflection of what's underneath. Keep it happy by nourishing your insides.

24

Strong Bones – Strong Body

Healthy bones are fundamental to good health. Unhealthy bones are more than just a concern – they can signify a significant decrease in structural integrity and raise red flags for overall health status. According to the International Osteoporosis Foundation,[1] a quarter of all men and fully half of all women will break at least one bone after the age of fifty. In both men and women, about half of those breaks will involve the hip. Hip fractures are especially deadly – a hip fracture triples the chances of dying within 5 years. In fact, one year after suffering a hip fracture, 20% of the victims will be dead, another 30% will be permanently disabled and at least 80% will not recover. Chronic back pain, loss of height, deformities, sleep disorders and mood problems are common consequences endured by survivors.

Maintaining healthy bone function entails several fundamentals of diet, lifestyle and nutritional support. While not difficult, incorporating these fundamentals to support optimal bone health is a meticulous process that requires life-long attention.

> *"…to support optimal bone health is a meticulous process that requires life-long attention."*

Nutrition and Bone Health

There have been a number of exciting discoveries in the 21st century that have expanded this relationship far beyond "drink more milk." Some well-known nutrients are becoming better understood and a few somewhat unexpected roles have been uncovered as the effects of the immune response on bones have begun to become appreciated. Excellent dietary practices (and a little help from bone-friendly supplements) and you'll be standing tall for decades to come.

Hot Tips for Better Bone Building

Calcium and Vitamin D – never alone, always together

The bedrock of every bone is an excellent supply of **calcium** and **vitamin D**. It's only logical – the hard substance of a bone is mostly calcium and vitamin D is needed in order for the gut to absorb calcium and for the bones to know what to do with it. Vitamin D regulates the body's calcium metabolism (and does much more). The importance of vitamin D for health is no longer a theory. It's a scientific fact. Its importance for bone health in conjunction with calcium is also well-established.

The results of three "gold standard" randomized placebo-controlled clinical trials all have shown that dietary supplementation with calcium promotes healthy bone structure. In one of these studies, elderly postmenopausal women without previous fractures responded to 4 years of daily dietary supplementation with 1000 mg of calcium with enhanced bone density and structure when compared to similar women being fed a placebo.[2] Similarly, a second study showed that elderly postmenopausal women who had previously suffered a spontaneous bone fracture, and had a lifetime of poor calcium nutrition prior to the study, responded to 4 years of daily dietary supplementation with 1200 mg of calcium with 77% fewer new spinal fractures than occurred in women fed a placebo for the 4 years.[3] In the third randomized placebo-controlled study, women who previously had suffered multiple fractures and then supplemented their diets with 1500 mg to 2500 mg of calcium daily also enjoyed fewer new fractures than were endured by similar women fed a placebo.[4]

The U.S. Food and Drug Administration has recognized the relationship between good calcium nutrition and bone health by stating that "Adequate calcium throughout life, as part of a well-balanced diet, may reduce the risk of osteoporosis." These government scientists continue to consider the significant scientific evidence that indicates that maintaining adequate calcium intake (that is, the amount that they recommend be consumed on a regular daily basis) can reduce the chances of suffering a spontaneous, "osteoporotic" fracture of the hip, spine or wrist.

A possible side-benefit of maintaining adequate calcium nutrition: On October 12, 2005, the U.S. Food and Drug Administration announced that although they found the scientific evidence inconsistent and not yet conclusive, they agreed that "Some scientific evidence suggests that calcium supplements may reduce the risk of hypertension."

Another possible side-benefit of maintaining adequate calcium nutrition: On October 12, 2005, the U.S. Food and Drug Administration announced that although the supporting scientific evidence is sparse and not conclusive, "Some evidence suggests that calcium supplements may reduce the risk of colon/rectal cancer" and "Very limited and preliminary evidence suggests that calcium supplements may reduce the risk of colon/rectal polyps."

But please do not think about calcium in isolation. The ability of calcium to benefit your bones (and cardiovascular system and digestive tract) depends on the cooperation of vitamin D. Unfortunately, even if you are making sure to get the recommended amount of vitamin D every single day, you still may not be getting enough vitamin D to optimally support your health.

What is the "Real" Vitamin D Requirement?

The true test of vitamin D adequacy is whether it prevents the parathyroid glands from secreting parathyroid hormone (PTH). What does the scientific evidence say? Daily intakes of vitamin D much greater than the recommended 400 IU are required to minimize PTH secretion and optimize skeletal health. The results of a statistical analysis of published research published recently in the *Journal of the American Medical Association* (*JAMA*) found that men and women over 60 years of age who routinely consumed double the RDA (about 800 IU of vitamin D daily) suffered 25% fewer hip fractures than those who stuck to the RDA.[5] Consistent with this analysis, the results of the Women's Health Initiative Study published recently in the *New England Journal of Medicine* proved that the RDA for vitamin D was no better than vitamin D deficient diets in protecting the skeleton.[6] As shown in the results of another study published recently in the *British Medical Journal*, even 800 IU daily may not be enough vitamin D for every elderly person.[7]

Scientists now conclude that an average vitamin D intake of 1000 IU daily is needed by most adults (some may require more) and that an average daily vitamin D intake of 2600 IU would be required in order to ensure that very few older women could become functionally vitamin D deficient. A pioneer of vitamin D research, Dr. Hector F. DeLuca of the University of Wisconsin, has advised all adults to consume 2000 IU of vitamin D daily to optimize health.[8] As detailed in the vitamin D chapter later on in this book, many researchers feel that a number of people may need much higher amounts. The FDA also agrees about the importance of achieving adequate intake of vitamin D along with calcium throughout life. In a claim they've approved about the relationship between vitamin D and calcium together, they state that, "Adequate calcium and vitamin

> "Calcium is the structural backbone for skeletal health and vitamin D controls its incorporation into tissues."

D throughout life, as part of a well-balanced diet, may reduce the risk of osteoporosis." Calcium is the structural backbone for skeletal health and vitamin D controls its incorporation into tissues. Both are vital to promoting healthy bone structure and density.

Vitamin C

Collagen is the major structural protein in bone. The proper synthesis and linking of collagen fibers requires large amounts of **vitamin C**. It is not surprising that nutritionists have found that the density and strength of adult bones increases as daily vitamin C intake increases.[9,10] With so many other ways to benefit from a regular intake of vitamin C, why take chances with your bones?

Phosphorus

The mineral **phosphorus** is as important to bone health as calcium. However, calcium and phosphorus sit on opposing sides of the mineral balance upon which your bones depend. Although phosphorus plays very critical roles in proving "attachment" sites for calcium in the mineral-dense areas of bone, it can compete with calcium for "room" in the blood. In other words, as the amount of phosphorus in the blood increases, the kidneys send more calcium out of the body. If your usual condition is too much phosphorus in your blood, then there will usually be too little calcium circulating through your body and the parathyroid gland will spark into action. As your bones are dissolved in the futile attempt to restore your blood's calcium content, the high level of phosphorus keeps on stimulating the kidney to shoot calcium back out – a bad situation for your skeleton. Because most people in North America habitually tend to consume foods and beverages that provide enormous amounts of phosphorus, restraint rather than supplementation is the key to healthy phosphorus nutrition.

Magnesium

Next to calcium and phosphorus, magnesium is the third most important mineral in the human skeleton. The results of a study assessing the importance of magnesium for bone health found that higher intakes of this mineral from the diet and dietary supplements was a predictor of higher bone mineral density in white males and females.[11] The large study assessed 2,038 men and women aged between 70 and 79 years of age. Again, no surprise: the density and strength of adult bones increases as daily magnesium intake increases.

Boron

A trace mineral that is found within bone, boron is yet to be assigned a specific function in maintaining bone health. However, rats fed a boron-free diet develop weak bones. The possible dependency of bone health on boron may be explained by reports that boron supplementation (3 mg daily) increased the conversion of vitamin D to 25-hydroxyvitamin D3 (25-OHD3) in women and that boron may be required for maximum efficiency in the absorption of calcium. An unanticipated relationship between boron, vitamin D and calcium absorption could account for the report that attributed maintenance of higher bone mineral density in women to daily dietary supplementation with 3 mg of boron.[12]

Fish Oils

Relationships between dietary fatty acids and bone health are only recently becoming appreciated. A role for the **fish oils** in bone certainly is suggested by their appearance within bone tissue. In the presence of the fatty acid eicosapentaenoic acid (EPA), bone cells display a healthy normalization of the immune response and secrete less of the bone resorption-promoting prostaglandin E_2 (PGE_2) when stimulated by the chemical messenger interleukin-1. Feeding rats fish oils decreases the rate of bone loss that results experimentally from a calcium-deficient diet. The bone mineral density of the hip in men and of the hip and spine in women were reported to be directly proportional to the average daily intake of fish oils.[13] Although the results of dietary supplementation studies in humans have not yet been reported, the available evidence all points toward an important bone health-enhancing effect of fish oils.

Saturated Fat

In most areas of human health, whenever fish oils are beneficial, saturated animal fats are detrimental. Your bones are no exception. As shown by the results of a study of 14,850 men and women (part of the National Health and Nutrition Examination Survey III) the more saturated fat that is consumed every day, the weaker the bones of the hip become.[14] The bone-weakening effects of saturated fatty acids may result from the tendency of this type of fat to increase inflammation, both locally within the hip and systemically throughout the body. This finding is in line with everything else that is known about saturated fats, which as a body of evidence encourages you to reduce your consumption of these generally unhealthy fats.

> "The bone-weakening effects of saturated fatty acids may result from the tendency of this type of fat to increase inflammation..."

Protein

A myth that still circulates in the world of nutrition is that eating large amounts of lean protein will increase calcium loss through the urine and predispose to osteoporosis. This has been proven to be a misconception and is just wrong. For example, when middle-aged men and women with a long history of fearful low-protein diets (providing less than 15% of total calories as protein) were fed either placebo or 55 g/day of a high quality animal meat protein in a study published recently in the *Journal of*

Endocrinology and Metabolism, the normalization of protein intake had *no* effect on urinary excretion of calcium but decreased bone resorption and increased the secretion of the cytokine, insulin-like growth factor-1 (IGF-1).[15] Because a major function of IGF-1 in adults is to stimulate bone formation, the combination of no effect on calcium loss, decreased bone resorption and stimulation of bone formation substantiate the conclusion that ensuring adequate healthy protein intake is truly beneficial to bone health. Of course, adequate protein intake is also beneficial for immune health, healthy blood sugar balance, and a number of other physiological effects.

This conclusion finds additional support in the results of a study published recently in the Annals of Surgery.[16] In this study, injections of human growth hormone were used to stimulate IGF-1 production and secretion into the blood. Increased serum IGF-1 concentrations were accompanied by increased total body bone mineral content. Because IGF-1 independently stimulates bone formation, this result indicates that any means that increases IGF-1 production, including increasing the daily intake of high-quality low-fat protein, will likely enhance bone health.

Soy Protein Isoflavones

Soy protein contains a set of phytochemicals called isoflavones. These phytonutrients are absorbed into the human blood stream and circulate to a variety of tissues where they interact with the processes regulating cell functions. One area of isoflavone biology that has received a great deal of attention is the support of bone health. Studies consistently show a beneficial effect of soy isoflavone consumption on human bone. The results of a hallmark randomized, placebo-controlled study demonstrated that several months of daily supplementation with 90 mg of soy isoflavones facilitated an increase in the bone mineral content and bone mineral density of the spine in postmenopausal women.[17] In contrast, only 56 mg daily was not effective. Another randomized, placebo-controlled study showed that daily consumption of 80 mg of soy isoflavones for 6 months supported the density of vertebral bone in perimenopausal women.[18] In confirmation of previous studies, two studies published recently demonstrated that less than 80 mg of soy isoflavones daily is ineffective in promoting bone health in postmenopausal women.[19,20]

Ipriflavone

In an effort to increase the effectiveness and acceptability of soy isoflavones, a modified isoflavone called ipriflavone was developed. When 600 mg of ipriflavone have been combined with 1000 mg of calcium daily, vertebral bone mass was enhanced in a group of postmenopausal women.[21]

Unfortunately, a shadow of doubt has been cast over the effectiveness of ipriflavone as a result of a misunderstanding of the results of a study published in the *Journal of the American Medical Association*.[22]. The results of that study showed pretty conclusively that if 600 mg of ipriflavone daily was combined with a dramatically calcium deficient diet (only 500 mg daily!), postmenopausal women still lost bone mass. Obviously, if the diet isn't sufficient in calcium, and therefore the body lacks calcium, bones are liable to be weak. Seems like a no-brainer, doesn't it? The correct message of this study is that if you want to improve bone health, no matter what you rely on to stimulate bone formation and slow resorption, enough calcium has to be available to make it work.

Vitamin K

Vitamin K is required for the production of the second most important protein (other than collagen) in bone – osteocalcin. This would suggest a connection between vitamin K intake and bone health. Indeed, human bone mineral density is proportional to vitamin K intake. This conclusion was confirmed and extended by the findings of an extensive analysis of published research that firmly suggested superior bone health with daily dietary supplementation of between 10 mcg and 45 mcg of vitamin K.[23]

Adults may have poor vitamin K status because 1) the widespread use of "blood-thinning" medications may interfere with this vitamin, 2) the primary dietary sources of vitamin K are the green leafy vegetables, which commonly are minimized in the North American diet, 3) more than dietary sources, humans rely on gut bacteria to produce vitamin K from dietary fiber, another often-avoided dietary necessity. The typical low-vegetable, low-fiber diet may be causing a form of undiagnosed vitamin K deficiency, manifested as impaired bone health.

The fear with excessive vitamin K intake is also the fact that vitamin K has interactions with blood clotting proteins. This is a valid concern for many individuals who are taking blood thinners and other medications. Recently, a form of supplemental vitamin K, known as menaquinone-7 (or MK-7), has come onto the dietary supplement scene. The menaquinones are a group of compounds that comprise the vitamin K2 family. MK-7 is much safer that vitamin K1 and possibly much more effective in supporting bone health. Several studies point to the beneficial effects of supplementation with vitamin K2 as MK-7. This form of vitamin K has health benefits beyond its important actions on bone, and may support cardiovascular and arterial health as well. MK-7 is naturally found in natto, a traditional fermented soy food consumed in Japan and some other Asian countries. With a better safety profile and superior health benefits, MK-7 should be considered a preferential supplemental form of vitamin K.

> *"...human bone mineral density is proportional to vitamin K intake."*

Exercise

Exercise is beneficial to bone health. "Use it or lose it" applies here – bones respond to loading and will increase their structural strength to meet gradually increasing demands. But, if never challenged, the failure point at which a bone will break instead of bend decreases, increasing the chances of incurring a spontaneous fracture.

The proof is in the data – volumes of it. For example, participation in regular physical activity more than ten hours a week cuts the chances of a man breaking a hip about in half. Women who exercise regularly have denser bones and less risk of developing osteoporosis. The degree of benefit depends on the duration and intensity of the activity – from the bones' points of view. The more the activity requires your skeleton to bear weight, the better. Weight-lifting is better than gymnastics, gymnastics is better than running, running is better than swimming and swimming beats sitting around.

There may be a fringe benefit to all this exercise. According to the results of a study published recently in *Europa Medicophysica*, regular controlled exercise improves spinal stability and decreases chronic low back pain.[24]

Enhancing bone health and structure requires a fundamental approach to establish habits that include several elements of a healthy skeletal support system. This approach encompasses dietary habits such as ensuring adequate protein intake, healthy amounts of calcium, and decreasing alcoholic and high phosphorus beverages, lifestyle approaches such as weight-bearing exercise, and smart supplementation with bone-building vitamins, minerals and other nutrients. By providing the bones with the building blocks they crave, you can ensure the structural support system of the body will remain stronger - longer.

25

Joint Health - Lubrication for your Hinges

Our mobility, flexibility, and independence all require joints that operate smoothly, efficiently and without a hitch. Even a slight amount of discomfort puts all of that in jeopardy. Most, if not all of us, have experienced some type of discomfort in our joints as a result of normal use, wear and tear, sports, our work or other activities. If not addressed early on, joint issues can become a constant source of worry later in life. Keeping our joints mobile, flexible and in tip-top shape, so that they recover from the rigors of our daily life quickly and efficiently, requires proper nutrition and providing them with the nutrients they need in the proper amounts. The correct foods and dietary supplements can add years of health to those vital links in your structure that are so important for a healthy, active lifestyle.

The emphasis of this chapter is to introduce the concept of maintaining joint health through nutritional choices we make on a daily basis. Several dietary choices and nutritional supplements that support healthy joints are discussed here. Elsewhere in the book, some of these nutrients are discussed in further detail as they pertain to joint health and other health benefits. Certain nutritional tactics are mentioned here for the first time because they are truly targeted to joint health. The benefits you can obtain from these nutritional sources are well-documented and in some cases universally acclaimed by nutritionists and physicians alike.

Hyaluronic Acid

Hyaluronic acid is a component found in normal, healthy joint tissue. As shown in research recently published in the *Journal of Physiology*, hyaluronic acid is responsible for keeping the joints hydrated – a property vital to the ability of joints to absorb shock and carry weight.[1] The slowdown in hyaluronic acid replenishment in joint cartilage that accompanies getting older can result in hyaluronic acid deficiency within a joint. Hyaluronic acid deficient joints become dry and lose their cushioning properties, predisposing them to a decrease in mobility.

Published scientific research has demonstrated that ensuring sufficient amounts of hyaluronic acid are available to your joints can promote joint health and function. The importance of the function of hyaluronic acid in joint tissue clearly substantiates the benefits of including it in your personal Joint Health program. See much more on hyaluronic acid in the dedicated chapter found later in the book.

> *"Hyaluronic acid is responsible for keeping the joints hydrated – a property vital to the ability of joints to absorb shock and carry weight."*

Fish Oils

Fish oils promote joint flexibility and ease of motion. In a study published recently in *Nutrition*, supplementation with 3000 mg of fish oils daily promoted healthy joint movement and flexibility in a group of middle-aged men.[2] This is just one example of the evidence that confirms the benefits that fish oils can provide to your joints. Recently, a meta-analysis of clinical studies concluded that consumption of fish oils led to the promotion of feelings of comfort and ease in the joints of individuals supplementing with them.[3] Fish oils play a vital role in supporting the recovery of joint comfort and function associated with everyday activities.

Glucosamine Sulfate

Glucosamine sulfate is another component of healthy joint cartilage that can be delivered to your joints through dietary supplementation. The results of 2 "gold standard," randomized double-blind placebo-controlled clinical trials have shown conclusively that men and women with mild to moderate degrees of joint discomfort and loss of flexibility experience clinically important improvements in joint ease and comfort, after a month of dietary supplementation with 1500 mg of daily glucosamine sulfate.[4,5] In addition, these improvements in joint characteristics are accompanied by increased ability to utilize the joint in daily activities - with minimal or no side effects – an important feature of any joint supportive therapy.

The results of two much longer randomized double-blind placebo-controlled clinical trials confirm the joint-friendly properties of glucosamine sulfate. In these two studies, 3 years of dietary supplementation with glucosamine sulfate (1500 mg/day) restored joint tissue and structure, and increased joint function while promoting joint comfort and mobility.[6,7] Various groups of investigators have concluded that daily dietary supplementation with 1500 mg of glucosamine sulfate for 6 weeks or more reduces joint discomfort and increases joint mobility, flexibility and ability to bear weight with excellent safety. The most recently completed systematic analysis concluded that 1500 mg of glucosamine sulfate daily is "effective and safe" in supporting knee joint

> "Glucosamine sulfate has been established as one of the foundational nutrients for promoting joint health as it is a key building block for strong healthy joints."

function and wellness.[8] Glucosamine sulfate has been established as one of the foundational nutrients for promoting joint health as it is a key building block for strong healthy joints.

Chondroitin Sulfate

Chondroitin sulfate is another key structural component of joint cartilage that works hand-in-hand with hyaluronic acid and glucosamine sulfate. Just like its two partners, chondroitin sulfate also has been shown repeatedly to enhance joint health and function. For example, in randomized, double-blind, placebo-controlled studies of subjects with joint discomfort due to various causes, dietary supplementation with chondroitin sulfate (1200 mg daily for 6 months) enhanced joint comfort and increased joint mobility, while also supporting the structural cushioning ability of cartilage tissue. Daily consumption of only 800 mg of chondroitin sulfate has been equally effective, although results were not apparent until after continuous supplementation for one year or more. Several groups of investigators have applied the techniques of meta-analysis to evaluate dietary supplementation with chondroitin sulfate. They have concluded that 1200 mg of chondroitin sulfate consumed daily for at least 4 months will produce noticeably improvements in joint comfort and function.[9-11] Chondroitin sulfate also has a high safety profile and fits the mold of being a core nutrient for joint wellbeing.

Type II Collagen

Supporting the body's immune response to various triggers affecting joint health can support the function of joints throughout the body. Enabling the immune system to become tolerant by exposing it to inactivated segments of type II collagen, the type of collagen found only in joints, may desensitize the response seen in cases of joint discomfort to the point where joints are no longer impacted and the body's overall inflammatory response is normalized. This is the theory that forms the basis for the beneficial effects associated with the administration of type II collagen as a joint health supplement.

Adults and adolescents alike have responded to dietary supplementation with 0.1 mg/day to 10 mg/day of various preparations of processed type II collagen with enhanced comfort and ease, and increased mobility in several joints. More impressively, the results of a randomized double-blind placebo-controlled clinical trial indicate that adults respond to 90 days of dietary supplementation with 0.5 mg of solubilized type II collagen daily with increased function, decreased sensations of pressure, and increased mobility.[13]

Vitamin C

Vitamin C is absolutely necessary for the production of strong collagen fibers, including those found within joint cartilage. Without adequate supplies of vitamin C, collagen fibers become weak and lose structural integrity. Mechanical failure of weakened joint cartilage can trigger joint discomfort and other joint health issues.

Data obtained from the 10-year prospective Iowa Women's Health Study of 29,368 women aged 55 years or older when the study began indicate that among these seemingly typical older US women, the chance of maintaining healthy joint structure and function among women consuming more than twice the current RDA for vitamin C was about twice as good as that among women consuming less vitamin C.[14] Consistent with this finding, other studies have found that routine daily vitamin C intakes greater than twice the current RDA enhance an individual's ability to maintain normal joint function with age.[15]

Boswellia serrata

Extracts of the herb *Boswellia serrata* may also provide support for maintaining a healthy immune balance within joints. In studies published recently in the *Journal of Ethnopharmacology*, *Boswellia serrata* extracts reduce the severity of experimentally induced joint conditions in animals by modulating the release of the immune system intercellular messenger cytokine, interleukin-1 .[16,17] By forcing the immune system to maintain the status quo, *Boswellia serrata* can aid in achieving comfortable, properly-functioning joints.

Stinging Nettle

Along with *Boswellia serrata*, research suggests that an extract of the stinging nettle plant may also promote a healthy, balanced immune response within joint tissue. According to the results of a human study published in the *Journal of the Royal Society of Medicine*, the extract of stinging nettle enhanced joint comfort in aching joints in older men and women.[18]

MSM (Methylsulfonylmethane)

MSM is an organic sulfur compound that is chemically inert. It occurs naturally in certain plants and is available as a dietary supplement for joint health. Sulfur is a mineral that is necessary for the health of connective tissue throughout the body, including the bones, joints, ligaments and tendons. Supplemental MSM provides sulfur that can be used in the formation and maintenance of these different types of connective tissue. Studies have shown that MSM can enhance joint health and function. Recently, a study conducted in India showed that MSM, alone and in combination with glucosamine, was able to promote joint comfort and mobility.[19] The study was a randomized double-blind placebo-controlled trial conducted in 118 individuals. Using MSM in combination with glucosamine, similar to the combination of glucosamine with chondroitin, may be another viable approach that nature has developed for helping us achieve functional, healthy joints.

Use Them, or Lose Them

There is something else you can do in addition to utilizing targeted nutrition to help your joints last as long as possible – exercise! Two recently published human studies have confirmed the roles of physical activity in joint health. A study published in the *Annals of the Rheumatic Diseases* showed that if you don't use your joints, their cartilage covering tends to thin out.[20] A second study published in the journal *Arthritis and Rheumatism* showed that moderate exercise increases the thickness of joint cartilage and improves joint performance.[21]

A combination of healthy dietary choices, supplemental nutrients, and exercise can lead to beneficial effects in terms of your ability to maintain optimal joint structure and integrity.

Section III

Healthy Habits - Developing a Plan that Fits Your Needs

Fundamentals of Healthy Aging

Habits of Highly Successful People

Aging is a process of gradual change that results in the accumulation of small incremental decreases in the normal functional capacities of the body and mind. Effects on outward appearance also become noticeable as changes occur in the skin, hair and nails. Other functional changes involve the regulation of metabolism and of physiological systems, affecting such things as immune function, vision, sexual performance, energy levels and sleep. Some of the changes that affect the body's structural elements – muscles, bones, joints, tendons and ligaments – occur gradually over many years. As these changes take place, movement, flexibility, strength, endurance and recovery from overuse or injury may be compromised. Also, because aging-associated changes can affect the body's control centers – the brain, spinal cord and nerves – cognitive functions, including memory formation and retrieval, quickness of thought, ability to concentrate and make decisions, attention span, emotional balance and mood – can become less reliable. Scientists have yet to agree upon a clear

> "Scientists have yet to agree upon a clear definition of aging, other than simply "getting older," but, like the rest of us, most know it when they see it."

definition of aging, other than simply "getting older," but, like the rest of us, most know it when they see it.

What Causes "Aging"?

Many theories abound for the causes of the signs of aging on the human body. A number of them make a certain amount of sense from a strictly empirical (that is, evidence-based) scientific point of view that focuses on the individual. A major theory is the "free radical theory of aging" that suggests that eventually the accumulation of the inevitable chemical imperfections in body biochemistry will cause enough damage to result in functional declines and failures in various body systems. The evidence for this is increasing, as we now know a number of physiological changes occur in cells throughout the body secondary to the ravages of oxidative stress. We also know that cells exposed to overwhelming oxidative damage eventually will succumb to it and die. It is also well-established that cells capable of defending themselves through the production or availability of antioxidant defenses can stay stronger, longer. Thus, according to this theory, the health of every cell, and thus organ, system and likely the human individual, is dependent on maintaining a balance that favors a higher amount of antioxidants to free radicals. Further evidence for this comes from studies showing that individuals consuming foods that are high in antioxidants, such as fruits and vegetables, generally are healthier overall than those individuals consuming diets low in antioxidant-rich foods. Based on these findings, it is easy to see how this theoretical perspective on the causes of aging has merit.

On the other hand, other theories attempt to explain the issue from larger perspectives, such as a sort of combination of environmental influences and genetic predetermination that lead to a determination of how cells, organs, systems and the body age. Studies of population groups comprising different ethnicities have shown that certain cultures certainly have varying genetic makeup and tendencies towards differing health concerns.

People in South Asia tend to have a greater incidence of heart disease than many other cultural groups throughout the world. Recently, genetic factors have been identified that likely explain this greater risk, at least in part. Several other such examples exist in cultures spanning the globe. In the end, all possibilities exert some influence on the process of "aging" and together combine to produce the changes in normal physiology associated with age.

The preceding can appear to describe an overwhelming situation – what some may describe as the "inevitability" of age. It's not surprising that so many people seem to surrender to these changes and choose to embrace "the inevitable." Please don't follow their example. They are not aware of and, therefore, cannot understand the key to "healthy aging" – for every dart that "growing older" seems to throw at you, Mother Nature offers you a shield. These shields, or principles, describe the foundations of healthy aging practices. Your job is to determine what those principles are, which principles apply to your individual case, and how to implement them in your daily life. Of course, if you've read through this book this far you know the answers. Now, the challenge is to actualize the principles that have been outlined here and incorporate them into your diet, your lifestyle practices, and your foundational nutritional regimen, adding to this foundation based on your own needs.

Is "Aging" Truly Inevitable?

Maybe not as we usually think of it. Evidence from a study published recently in the *Journal of Gerontology* points to some interesting facts about centenarians. Gerontologists evaluated the reports of 42,398 consecutive autopsies that were performed between 1975 and 1995 in Vienna, Austria. They found that 40 of these men and women were over the age of 100 years when they died. Of these 40, 24 (60%) were *completely healthy* when they died. All 40 were reported to have suffered an acute fatal heart attack or to have simply stopped breathing – none seemed to have died of "old age." From all appearances they could have kept on living if whatever triggered their final moments had not occurred. According to these specialists, while "getting older" is inevitable, "dying of old age" is not. Death may also be inevitable; however living healthfully by incorporating healthy practices can lead to "Healthy Aging". Most of the centenarians in this study seem to have found that "holy grail" of human health – they got older without being harmed by the experience.

What Is "Healthy Aging"?

Retaining true physical youth happens nowhere in nature and would be unnatural. That's why "anti-aging" is a misconception – "aging" cannot be prevented unless you have access to a working time machine. If you do, all bets are off. Otherwise, realize that fighting against "aging" is a fairly futile practice. Not even the Spanish conquistadors could find the Fountain of Youth. As someone once said, *"Aging seems to be the only available way to live a long life."*

> *"...while "getting older" is inevitable, "dying of old age" is not."*

"Healthy aging", therefore, is one part prevention of functional decline and one part extension of longevity. Thanks to today's understanding of the science of life, remaining as "youthful" as possible for as many decades as possible, with the fringe benefit of a few extra decades – now *that* is an achievable goal.

How Can It Be Achieved?

Population-based studies suggest that there are practices that healthy people around the world have implemented which show promise for living longer, healthier lives. In fact, a number of population groups around the world are living the "Healthy Aging" dream right now.

In Okinawa, Japan, over 600 men and women have exceeded a century of life and are still going strong (http://www.okicent.org/ study.html). It's not just a coincidence that Okinawa has higher than average numbers of centenarians; the average life expectancy of the 1.4 million Okinawans is almost 90 years. And they don't just live longer, they live better longer. Compared to men and women in the US, Okinawans more than 65 years old have about one-quarter the rate of loss of cognitive functioning, half as many hip fractures, one-fifth as much heart disease, half the rate of colon cancer, one-fifth as much breast cancer and only 10% as many cases of prostate cancer. Yet, so far as researchers can determine, there are no relevant "longevity-enhancing" genetic differences between North Americans and Okinawans. Can lifestyle and diet really be that important? You be the judge – going beyond the "outcomes" statistics quoted above, it is known that on average an Okinawan has less than half as many free radicals circulating in his or her blood as has a North American.

To recap: <u>live right, eat right, suffer half as much chronic oxidative stress, and enjoy a ten to twenty-year longer, and much more disease-free, lifespan.</u> Doesn't that sound motivating?

What are Okinawans Doing?

Several "themes" have become apparent when the lifestyles of the longest-lived Okinawans have been examined. Perhaps most importantly, they are not overweight. In fact, they tend to be slightly underweight – naturally! – they have enjoyed a lifetime of lean trimness without any periods of adult excess fat accumulation. In terms of dietary practices, their habit is to stop eating at the first feelings of fullness, instead of stuffing themselves with excess food. If you don't gain it you never need to lose it.

They begin life active and they remain in motion as much as is possible, exercising every day in the form of dance, soft martial arts, walking and gardening. They seem to embody a type of personification of that old physics adage that a body in motion tends to remain in motion and not collapse under its own inertia.

Of course, they also shun self-destructive use of tobacco products or alcohol to excess.

Personality testing has found that Okinawan centenarians, when they were decades younger and in their prime of life, scored low when it came to feelings of "time urgency" and "tension" and high in "self-confidence" and "unyieldingness." Interviews revealed optimistic attitudes, adaptability, and an easy-going approach to life. Moderation was found to be a key cultural value. Strong social integration and a deep spirituality were particularly evident among Okinawan women. These all tend to be habits and outlooks that contribute to a low-stress lifestyle. Stress being a major cause of disease, it's fruitful to avoid stress as much as possible - the Okinawan way of life.

What about in the Mediterranean?

In those areas where the Mediterranean dietary lifestyle is traditional, the people with the greatest health and longevity eat abundant amounts of fresh fruits and vegetables, fish, whole grain breads, beans, nuts, seeds, olives and olive oil, cheeses made from the milks of species other than cows and the occasional glass or two of red wine, a rich source of antioxidant compounds from grapes such as resveratrol, with a meal. Concentrated sugars, processed flour products, eggs, cheeses made from cow's milk, lean red meats and dairy products are considered rare treats.

Establishing Your "Healthy Aging" Plan

Learn From The Okinawans & The People Of The Mediterranean!

First and foremost – slow down. Relax a little. Definitely don't stress about it!

Now, take a leisurely but long and honest look at your lifestyle. While you're relaxing is a good time to ask yourself: Is the way I eat fostering "old age" or is it promoting Healthy Aging?

A sensible way to assess the contribution your nutritional practices are making to your ability to age healthfully is to compare them to the information you have learned from this book.

Then, in a stepwise fashion, think about making incremental changes to your habits that will lead you down the path of health and wellness. Think of the core elements that we've talked about time and again. These include the fundamentals of diet, lifestyle, and nutritional therapy. Now, thinking about each one, assess where you may be deficient and then give some thought to incorporating healthy principles into your daily living.

Taking it one step further, your therapeutic nutritional regimen should work as follows: the foundational nutrients should include a high-quality, complete multivitamin and multimineral formula that has sufficient levels of essential nutrients and includes additional antioxidants. Given the immense benefits of essential fatty acids from fish oil, these should be a part of the foundational plan. A high-potency, purified fish oil product is best. In addition to these supplements, a final one to include in this foundation is a probiotic bacterial supplement that contains multiple friendly strains and that is certified to contain what it states on the label.

> "...think about making incremental changes to your habits that will lead you down the path of health and wellness."

Now reassess your dietary habits and your lifestyle, along with any specific areas of need or support you have, and build on your foundation based on your needs. For example, if you're not getting adequate levels of antioxidants in your diet, you may need to add additional ones. This can be accomplished in many ways, including by adding a greens drink to your regimen. Furthermore, if you need to support your joints, cognitive function, or heart health, you would add nutrients specifically targeted to those areas. In this way, you start with the fundamental core of nutrients and then add based on your individual situation. This ensures you achieve the comprehensive support you are looking for in order to age healthfully. Lastly, if you need guidance, don't hesitate to check with your naturopathic physician or nutritionally-informed healthcare practitioner. It could be the wisest investment you'll ever make. So, if you need help, ask for it!

—*Tier I – Diet and Lifestyle*

Most of the food you eat should consist of fruits and vegetables as well as some whole grains (but not too many grain-based foods; they pack a sizeable caloric wallop). **Five servings of fruits and five servings of vegetables every day** will go a long way toward keeping you healthy. Eat a variety of fruits and vegetables – during the course of a week, your 35 servings of fruits should include at least 10 different kinds of fruit – go ahead and stretch your sense of adventure beyond apples, oranges and bananas. Eat some blueberries, fresh grapes, pineapple, papaya – you get the idea.

The same for vegetables – 35 servings a week, with 5 or fewer being any form of potatoes. Carrots, lettuce and tomatoes are great – but use your imagination. Replace a plate of fries with a bell pepper (green, red, yellow or orange) stuffed with mushrooms. Rotate different varieties of squash and zucchini. Cucumbers aren't just for sandwiches. And olives – how can you go wrong? Don't be afraid to actually try some of those "unusual" vegetables available in the stores. Eat a rainbow of colors, as those colors represent something healthy that your body has an essential need for.

Get adequate amounts of protein in your diet. Try to remember that the healthiest protein sources for human adults do not come from mammals. You've heard this before – fish every day, poultry several times a week and eggs as often as you like. View dairy foods (even the so-called "fat-free" ones) as beverages or sweet treats and not as components of a healthy diet. Eat very lean red meats on occasion to add some variety to meals, but don't fall into the "meat and potatoes" trap. And don't forget – beans and legumes are a great substitute for animal protein once in a while.

Snack on raw nuts and seeds as they are good sources of essential, healthy fats. Don't overdo it, though. They are calorie-rich.

Forget salt and sugar – you'll get all you need and then some from the fruits and vegetables that form the base of your relationship to food. Add spices to spice up your life – switch to some real taste enhancers – herbs, spices such as turmeric, ginger, coriander, cayenne, cinnamon, pepper – condiments that taste great, are less filling and are health-promoting.

Lastly, don't forget the importance of establishing a routine regimen of physical activity and exercise. Alternate this with a spiritual practice or some form of meditation, such as yoga. These routines will help you cope with daily stress.

—Tier II – Your Nutrition Insurance Policy

Of course, day-to-day life has its ups and downs, and it's not realistic to plan on always being able to keep up with your dietary ideals, no matter how motivated and well-intentioned you may be. Besides, there's no way you can maximize your nutritional health through foods alone – you just can't eat a dozen oranges, snack on a bushel of wild berries or wolf down 5 pounds of even the tastiest broiled salmon every day. Or even every other day. Also realize that the nutritional value of our foods has decreased over the years due to irregularities in soil nutrient content, over-planting and over-harvesting.

In the real world, everyone needs a nutritional insurance policy – and individualized, carefully selected and targeted high-quality dietary supplements are the answer.

As we discussed above, the "basic" policy is provided by a superior multivitamin, multimineral supplement. Daily use will smooth out the fluctuations in your needs and food choices and can fill in any temporary gaps that might occur on any particular day.

> *"...everyone needs a nutritional insurance policy – and individualized, carefully selected and targeted high-quality dietary supplements are the answer."*

You can use this book as a guide to what to look for. In general, a superior vitamin and mineral supplement for an adult should provide:

- Vitamin A
- Riboflavin
- Biotin
- Pantothenic acid
- Vitamin B12
- Vitamin D
- Vitamin K
- Chromium
- Magnesium
- Selenium
- Potassium

- Thiamin
- Niacin
- Folic Acid
- Vitamin B6
- Vitamin C
- Vitamin E
- Calcium
- Iodine
- Zinc
- Molybdenum

In addition to a superior multivitamin and multimineral supplement, you should add supplemental fish oil and a probiotic supplement. Quality products are essential to ensure you're getting all of the good they offer and none of the bad - in terms of contamination, rancidity, certified strains, etc.

Beyond that, give consideration to adding a "whole foods" dietary supplement containing fruit and vegetable extracts or powders, if your dietary habits haven't reached the healthy plateau yet. A fun and refreshing alternative is a "whole foods" liquid beverage packed with all of these nutrients plus a broad spectrum of phytochemicals, the dietary fiber of fruits and vegetables, and the other, so far unidentified, healthy food factors that nicely complement the purified vitamins and minerals in your basic supplement. A couple of these drinks a day can make up for any servings of fruits or vegetables you might happen to miss.

—Tier III – Individualize and Target Your Coverage

The judicious selection and then faithful consumption of other dietary supplementation will allow you to focus on your greatest personal concerns. Want extra immune support? A concentrated bioflavonoid mix may be helpful. Joint support? Think glucosamine, chondroitin sulfate, hyaluronic acid, etc. If heart health concerns you, you may want to include CoQ10 and alpha-lipoic acid, among others in your daily "Tier III" supplemental nutrition plan for Healthy Aging. Looking for an edge in mental performance, memory, mental clarity, quick thinking? Consider folic acid, the omega-3 fish oils EPA and DHA, dark green leafy vegetables, blueberries, phosphatidylserine, *N*-acetylcysteine, vinpocetine and other brain-friendly phytonutrients.

Need help deciding? The chapters of this book are designed to assist you. For further guidance, consult a naturopathic physician or nutritionally-oriented health care practitioner.

Despite what you may want to think, it is impossible to take every supplement that could help improve your health. That's why the basis of your nutrition plan for Healthy Aging is healthy food choices. Your dietary habits are of the utmost importance. Nonetheless, everyone can benefit from first identifying their own most urgent needs and then targeting their personalized nutrition plan for Healthy Aging accordingly.

Healthy Aging – Go For It!

Although Mark Twain said, "The only way to keep your health is to eat what you don't want, drink what you don't like, and do what you'd druther not," when you embrace a positive lifestyle – eating healthfully, exercising moderately and joyfully filled with a sense of purpose, passion and social engagement – you will find that *Healthy Aging* is a journey well worth pursuing.

A Blueprint for Healthy Aging

- A healthy diet is the foundation of healthy aging.
- Fill in the gaps with individualized and targeted dietary supplementation.
- Build on that core with daily physical activity and exercise.

- Never use tobacco products and drink red wine at dinner and in moderation.
- Embrace your life as it is, and let a desire to improve – not ambition – guide you.
- Become inspired by whatever makes you truly happy and fulfilled
- Turn your back on stress and learn to relax.
- Turn toward the meaningful people in your life and allow their love and friendship to restore your energy.
- Rekindle your trust in others.
- Exercise your mind and challenge it to retain a positive outlook and attitude.
- Laugh once in a while and smile often.
- Maintain balance in all things.

References

Chapter 1

1. Harris WS, Sands SA, Windsor SL, Ali HA, Stevens TL, Mgalski A, Porter CB, Borkon AM. Omega-3 fatty acids in cardiac biopsies from heart transplantation patients. Correlation with erythrocytes and response to supplementation. *Circulation* 2004;110:1645-1649.
2. Hill AM, Buckley JD, Murphy KJ, Howe PR. Combining fish-oil supplements with regular aerobic exercise improves body composition and cardiovascular disease risk factors. *Am J Clin Nutr.* 2007;85(5):1267-74.
3. Christensen JH, Christensen MS, Dyerberg J, Schmidt EB. Heart rate variability and fatty acid content of blood cell membranes: A dose-response study with n-3 fatty acids. *Am J Clin Nutr* 1999;70:331-337.
4. Holguin F, Tellez-Rojo MM, Lazo M, Mannino D, Schwartz J, Hernandez M, Romieu I. Cardiac autonomic changes associated with fish oil vs soy oil supplementation in the elderly. *Chest* 2005;127:1102-1107.
5. Geelen A, Zock PL, Swenne CA, Brouwer IA, Schouten EG, Katan MB. Effect of n-3 fatty acids on heart rate variability and baroreflex sensitivity in middle-aged subjects. *Am Heart J* 2003;146:e4.
6. Christensen JH, Gustenhoff P, Korup E, Aaroe J, Toft E, Moller J, Rasmussen K, Dyerberg J, Schmidt EB. Effect of fish oil on heart rate variability in survivors of myocardial infarction: A double blind randomised controlled trial. *BMJ* 1996;312:677-678.
7. Mozaffarian D, Geelen A, Brouwer IA, Geleijnse JM, Zock PL Katan MB. Effect of fish oil on heart rate in humans. A meta-analysis of randomized controlled trials. *Circulation* 2005;112:1945-1952.
8. von Schacky C, Angerer P, Kothny W, Theisen K, Mudra H. The effect of dietary omega-3 fatty acids on coronary atherosclerosis. A randomized, double-blind, placebo-controlled trial. *Ann Intern Med* 1999;130:554-562.
9. Faeh D, Minehira K, Schwarz JM, Periasamy R, Park S, Tappy L. Effect of fructose overfeeding and fish oil administration on hepatic de novo lipogenesis and insulin sensitivity in healthy men. *Diabetes* 2005;54:1907-1913.
10. Dallongeville J, Yarnell J, Ducimetiere P, Arveiler D, Ferrieres J, Montaye M, Luc G, Evans A, Bingham A, Hass B, Ruidavets JB, Amouyel P. Fish consumption is associated with lower heart rates. *Circulation* 2003;108:820-825.
11. Nestel P, Shige H, Pomeroy S, Cehun M, Abbey M, Raederstorff D. The n-3 fatty acids eicosapentaenoic acid and docosahexaenoic acid increase systemic arterial compliance in humans. *Am J Clin Nutr* 2002;76:326-330.
12. Institute of Medicine. Macronutrients and healthful diets. In: Panel on Macronutrients, Panel on the Definition of Dietary

Fiber, Subcommittee on Upper Reference Levels of Nutrients, Subcommittee on Interpretation and Uses of Dietary Reference Intakes, and the Standing Committee on the Scientific Evaluation of Dietary Reference Intakes. *Dietary Reference Intakes for Energy, Carbohydrate, Fiber, Fat, Fatty Acids, Cholesterol, Protein, and Amino Acids (Macronutrients)*. The National Academies Press, Washington, DC, 2005, pp. 769-879.

13. Crawford MA. The early development and evolution of the human brain. *Ups J Med Sci Suppl.* 1990;48:43-78.

14. Parasuraman R, Greenwood PM, Kumar R, Fossella J. Beyond heritability: Neurotransmitter genes differentially modulate visuospatial attention and working memory. *Psychol Sci* 2005;16:200-207.

15. Whalley LJ, Fox HC, Wahle KW, Starr JM, Deary IJ. Cognitive aging, childhood intelligence, and the use of food supplements: Possible involvement of n-3 fatty acids. *Am J Clin Nutr* 2004;80:1650-1657.

16. Morris MC, Evans DA, Tangney CC, Bienias JL, Wilson RS. Fish consumption and cognitive decline with age in a large community study. *Arch Neurol* 2005;62:1849-1853.

17. Kalmijn S, van Boxtel MP, Ocke M, Verschuren WM, Kromhout D, Launer LJ. Dietary intake of fatty acids and fish in relation to cognitive performance at middle age. *Neurology* 2004;62:275-280.

18. Johnson EJ, Schaefer EJ. Potential role of dietary n-3 fatty acids in the prevention of dementia and macular degeneration. *Am J Clin Nutr.* 2006;83(6 Suppl):1494S-1498S.

19. 20. Tiemeier H, van Tuijl HR, Hofman A, Kiliaan AJ, Breteler MM. Plasma fatty acid composition and depression are associated in the elderly: The Rotterdam Study. *Am J Clin Nutr* 2003;78:40-46.

21. Peet M. International variations in the outcome of schizophrenia and the prevalence of depression in relation to national dietary practices: An ecological analysis. *Br J Psychiatry* 2004;184:404-408.

22. Nemets H, Nemets B, Apter A, Bracha Z, Belmaker RH. Omega-3 treatment of childhood depression: a controlled, double-blind pilot study. *Am J Psychiatry.* 2006;163(6):1098-100.

23. Rotstein NP, Politi LE, German OL, Girotti R. Protective effect of docosahexaenoic acid on oxidative stress-induced apoptosis of retina photoreceptors. *Invest Ophthalmol Vis Sci* 2003;44:2252-2259.

24. Chong EW, Kreis AJ, Wong TY, Simpson JA, Guymer RH. Dietary omega-3 fatty acid and fish intake in the primary prevention of age-related macular degeneration: a systematic review and meta-analysis. *Arch Ophthalmol.* 2008;126(6):826-33.

25. Ferrucci L, Cherubini A, Bandinelli S, Bartali B, Corsi A, Lauretani F, Martin A, Andres-Lacueva C, Senin U, Guralnik JM. Relationship of plasma polyunsaturated fatty acids to circulating inflammatory markers. *J Clin Endocrinol Metab* 2006;91:439-446.

26. Boelsma E, Hendriks HF, Roza L. Nutritional skin care: Health effects of micronutrients and fatty acids. *Am J Clin Nutr* 2001;73:853-864.

27. Chapkin RS, Ziboh VA, Marcelo CL, Voorhees JJ. Metabolism of

essential fatty acids by human epidermal enzyme preparations: Evidence of chain elongation. *J Lipid Res* 1986;27:945-954.

28. Berbert AA, Kondo CR, Almendra CL, Matsuo T, Dichi I. Supplementation of fish oil and olive oil in patients with rheumatoid arthritis. *Nutrition* 2005;21:131-136.

29. von Schacky C, Harris WS. Cardiovascular benefits of omega-3 fatty acids. *Cardiovascular Research* 2006; August (doi: 10.1016/j. cardiores.2006.08.019).

30. Foran JA, Good DH, Carpenter DO, Hamilton MC, Knuth BA, Schwager SJ. Quantitative analysis of the benefits and risks of consuming farmed and wild salmon. *J Nutr* 2005;135:2639-2643.

31. Helland IB, Smith L, Saarem K, Saugstad OD, Drevon CA Maternal supplementation with very-long-chain n-3 fatty acids during pregnancy and lactation augments children's IQ at 4 years of age. *Pediatrics* 2003;111:e39-e44.

32. Oken E, Wright RO, Kleinman KP, Bellinger D, Amarasiriwardena CJ, Hu H, Rish-Edwards JW, Gillman MW. Maternal fish consumption, hair mercury, and infant cognition in a U.S. cohort. *Environ Health Perspect* 2005;113:1376-1380.

Chapter 2

1. Cannell JJ, Hollis BW, Sorenson MB, Taft TN, Anderson JJ. Athletic Performance and Vitamin D. *Med Sci Sports Exerc.* 2009; 41(5):1102-1110.

2. Cannell JJ, Hollis BW. Use of vitamin D in clinical practice. *Altern Med Rev* 2008 Mar;13(1):6-20.

3. Heaney RP, Armas LA, Shary JR, Bell NH, Binkley N, Hollis BW. 25-Hydroxylation of vitamin D3: relation to circulating vitamin D3 under various input conditions. *Am J Clin Nutr.* 2008; 87(6):1738-42.

4. Aloia JF, Patel M, Dimaano R, Li-Ng M, Talwar SA, Mikhail M, Pollack S, Yeh JK. Vitamin D intake to attain a desired serum 25-hydroxyvitamin D concentration. *Am J Clin Nutr.* 2008 Jun;87(6):1952-8.

5. Calvo MS, Whiting SJ. Overview of the proceedings from Experimental Biology 2004 symposium: Vitamin D insufficiency: A significant risk factor in chronic diseases and potential disease-specific biomarkers of vitamin D sufficiency. *J Nutr* 2005;135:301-303.

6. Holick MF. Vitamin D: importance in the prevention of cancers, type 1 diabetes, heart disease, and osteoporosis. *Am J Clin Nutr* 2004;79:362-371.

7. Holick MF, Siris ES, Binkley N, Beard MK, Khan A, Katzer JT, Petruschke RA, Chen E, de Papp AE. Prevalence of Vitamin D inadequacy among postmenopausal North American women receiving osteoporosis therapy. *J Clin Endocrinol Metab* 2005;90:3215-

3224.
8. Hanley DA, Davison KS. Vitamin D insufficiency in North America. *J Nutr* 2005;135:332-337.
9. Moore CE, Murphy MM, Holick MF. Vitamin D intakes by children and adults in the United States differ among ethnic groups. *J Nutr* 2005;135:2478-2485.
10. Harris SS. Vitamin D and African Americans. *J Nutr* 2006;136:1126-1129.
11. Hollis BW. Circulating 25-hydroxyvitamin D levels indicative of vitamin D sufficiency: Implications for establishing a new effective dietary intake recommendation for vitamin D. *J Nutr* 2005;135:317-322.
12. Hashemipour S, Larijani B, Adibi H, Sedaghat M, Pajouhi M, Bastan-Hagh MH, Soltani A, Javadi E, Shafaei AR, Baradar-Jalili R, Hossein-Nezhad A. The status of biochemical parameters in varying degrees of vitamin D deficiency. *J Bone Miner Metab* 2006;24:213-218.
13. Steingrimsdottir L, Gunnarsson O, Indridason OS, Franzson L, Sigurdsson G. Relationship between serum parathyroid hormone levels, vitamin D sufficiency, and calcium intake. *JAMA* 2005;294:2336-2341.
14. Snijder MB, van Schoor NM, Pluijm SM, van Dam RM, Visser M, Lips P. Vitamin D status in relation to one-year risk of recurrent falling in older men and women. *J Clin Endocrinol Metab* 2006;91:2980-2985.
15. Bischoff-Ferrari HA, Willett WC, Wong JB, Giovannucci E, Dietrich T, Dawson-Hughes B. Fracture prevention with vitamin D supplementation: A meta-analysis of randomized controlled trials. *JAMA* 2005;293:2257-2264.
16. Jackson RD, LaCroix AZ, Gass M, Wallace RB, Robbins J, Lewis CE, Bassford T, Beresford SA, Black HR, Blanchette P, Bonds DE, Brunner RL, Brzyski RG, Caan B, Cauley JA, Chlebowski RT, Cummings SR, Granek I, Hays J, Heiss G, Hendrix SL, Howard BV, Hsia J, Hubbell FA, Johnson KC, Judd H, Kotchen JM, Kuller LH, Langer RD, Lasser NL, Limacher MC, Ludlam S, Manson JE, Margolis KL, McGowan J, Ockene JK, O'Sullivan MJ, Phillips L, Prentice RL, Sarto GE, Stefanick ML, Van Horn L, Wactawski-Wende J, Whitlock E, Anderson GL, Assaf AR, Barad D; Women's Health Initiative Investigators. Calcium plus vitamin D supplementation and the risk of fractures. *N Engl J Med* 2006;354:669-683.
17. Porthouse J, Cockayne S, King C, Saxon L, Steele E, Aspray T, Baverstock M, Birks Y, Dumville J, Francis R, Iglesias C, Puffer S, Sutcliffe A, Watt I, Torgerson DJ. Randomised controlled trial of calcium and supplementation with cholecalciferol (vitamin D3) for prevention of fractures in primary care. *BMJ* 2005;330:1003 (6 pages). doi:10.1136/bmj.330.7498.1003 (http://bmj.com/cgi/content/full/330/7498/1003).
18. DeLuca HF. Overview of general physiologic features and functions of vitamin D. *Am J Clin Nutr* 2004;80(Suppl.):1689S-1696S.
19. Pittas AG, Dawson-Hughes B, Li T, Van Dam RM, Willett WC,

Manson JE, Hu FB. Vitamin D and calcium intake in relation to type 2 diabetes in women. *Diabetes Care* 2006;29:650-656.

20. Giovannucci E, Liu Y, Rimm EB, Hollis BW, Fuchs CS, Stampfer MJ, Willett WC. Prospective study of predictors of vitamin D status and cancer incidence and mortality in men. *J Natl Cancer Inst* 2006;98:451-459.

21. Grau MV, Baron JA, Sandler RS, Haile RW, Beach ML, Church TR, Heber D. Vitamin D, calcium supplementation, and colorectal adenomas: Results of a randomized trial. *J Natl Cancer Inst* 2003;95:1765-1771.

22. Wactawski-Wende J, Kotchen JM, Anderson GL, Assaf AR, Brunner RL, O'Sullivan MJ, Margolis KL, Ockene JK, Phillips L, Pottern L, Prentice RL, Robbins J, Rohan TE, Sarto GE, Sharma S, Stefanick ML, Van Horn L, Wallace RB, Whitlock E, Bassford T, Beresford SA, Black HR, Bonds DE, Brzyski RG, Caan B, Chlebowski RT, Cochrane B, Garland C, Gass M, Hays J, Heiss G, Hendrix SL, Howard BV, Hsia J, Hubbell FA, Jackson RD, Johnson KC, Judd H, Kooperberg CL, Kuller LH, LaCroix AZ, Lane DS, Langer RD, Lasser NL, Lewis CE, Limacher MC, Manson JE; Women's Health Initiative Investigators. Calcium plus vitamin D supplementation and the risk of colorectal cancer. *N Engl J Med* 2006;354:684-696.

23. Chen L, Cencioni MT, Angelini DF, Borsellino G, Battistini L, Brosnan CF. Transcriptional profiling of T cells identifies a role for vitamin D in the immunoregulation of the V 9V 2 response to phosphate-containing ligands. *J Immunol* 2005;174:6144-6152.

24. Wang T-T, Nestel FP, Bourdeau V, Nagai Y, Wang Q, Liao J, Tavera-Mendoza L, Lin R, Hanrahan JH, Mader S, White JH. Cutting edge: 1,25-Dihydroxyvitamin D_3 is a direct inducer of antimicrobial peptide gene expression. J Immunol 2004;173:2909-2912.

25. Gombart AF, Borregaard N, Koeffler HP. Human cathelicidin antimicrobial peptide (CAMP) gene is a direct target of the vitamin D receptor and is strongly up-regulated in myeloid cells by 1,25-dihydroxyvitamin D3. *FASEB J* 2005;19:1067-1077.

26. Liu PT, Stenger S, Li H, Wenzel L, Tan BH, Krutzik SR, Ochoa MT, Schauber J, Wu K, Meinken C, Kamen DL, Wagner M, Bals R, Steinmeyer A, Zugel U, Gallo RL, Eisenberg D, Hewison M, Hollis BW, Adams JS, Bloom BR, Modlin RL. Toll-like receptor triggering of a vitamin D-mediated human antimicrobial response. *Science* 2006;311:1770-1773.

27. Pedrosa MAC, Moreira LDF, Barros ER, Kunii I, Lazaretti-Castro M. Cholecalciferol supplementation reverts 25-hydroxyvitamin D (25OHD) insufficiency and increases lower limb muscle strength (LLMS) in elderly people living in long-stay geriatric care (LSGC) (abstract P367SA). *Proceedings, International Osteoporosis Foundation World Congress on Osteoporosis*, Toronto, Canada, June 2-6, 2006, pp. 132-133.

Chapter 3

1.   Jeong YJ, Choi YJ, Kwon HM, Kang SW, Park HS, Lee M, Kang YH. Differential inhibition of oxidized LDL-induced apoptosis in human endothelial cells treated with different flavonoids. *Br J Nutr* 2005;93:581-591.

2.   Bu L, Lephart ED. AVPV neurons containing estrogen receptor-beta in adult male rats are influenced by soy isoflavones. *BMC Neurosci* 2007 Feb 1;8:13 (doi:10.1186/1471-2202-8-13).

3.   Santangelo C, Varì R, Scazzocchio B, Di Benedetto R, Filesi C, Masella R. Polyphenols, intracellular signalling and inflammation. *Ann Ist Super Sanita*. 2007;43(4):394-405. Review.

4.   Arts IC, Hollman PC. Polyphenols and disease risk in epidemiologic studies. *Am J Clin Nutr* 2005;81(Suppl.):317S-325S.

5.   Peluso MR. Flavonoids attenuate cardiovascular disease, inhibit phosphodiesterase, and modulate lipid homeostasis in adipose tissue and liver. *Exp Biol Med* 2006;231:1287-1299.

6.   Suh N, Paul S, Hao X, Simi B, Xiao H, Rimando AM, Reddy BS. Pterostilbene, an active constituent of blueberries, suppresses aberrant crypt foci formation in the azoxymethane-induced colon carcinogenesis model in rats. *Clin Cancer Res* 2007;13:350-355.

7.   Joseph JA, Shukitt-Hale B, Casadesus G. Reversing the deleterious effects of aging on neuronal communication and behavior: Beneficial properties of fruit polyphenolic compounds. *Am J Clin Nutr* 2005;81(Suppl.):313S-316S.

8.   Andres-Lacueva C, Shukitt-Hale B, Galli RL, Jauregui O, Lamuela-Raventos RM, Joseph JA. Anthocyanins in aged blueberry-fed rats are found centrally and may enhance memory. *Nutr Neurosci* 2005;8:111-120.

9.   Lau FC, Bielinski DF, Joseph JA. Inhibitory effects of blueberry extract on the production of inflammatory mediators in lipopolysaccharide-activated BV2 microglia. *J Neurosci Res* 2007 Jan 30 (doi: 10.1002/jnr.21205).

10. Duffy KB, Spangler EL, Devan BD, Guo Z, Bowker JL, Janas AM, Hagepanos A, Minor RK, DeCabo R, Mouton PR, Shukitt-Hale B, Joseph JA, Ingram DK. A blueberry-enriched diet provides cellular protection against oxidative stress and reduces a kainate-induced learning impairment in rats. *Neurobiol Aging*. 2008;29(11):1680-9.

11. Yang JH, Hsia TC, Kuo HM, Chao PD, Chou CC, Wei YH, Chung JG. Inhibition of lung cancer cell growth by quercetin glucuronides via G2/M arrest and induction of apoptosis. *Drug Metab Dispos* 2006;34:296-304.

12. Lu X, Jung J, Cho HJ, Lim DY, Lee HS, Chun HS, Kwon DY, Park JH. Fisetin inhibits the activities of cyclin-dependent kinases leading to cell cycle arrest in HT-29 human colon cancer cells. *J Nutr* 2005;135:2884-2890.

13. Murray TJ, Yang X, Sherr DH. Growth of a human mammary tumor cell line is blocked by galangin, a naturally occurring bioflavonoid,

and is accompanied by down-regulation of cyclins D3, E, and A. *Breast Cancer Res* 2006;8:R1 (doi: 10.1186/bcr1391).

14. Maher P, Akaishi T, Abe K. Flavonoid fisetin promotes ERK-dependent long-term potentiation and enhances memory. *Proc Natl Acad Sci U S A* 2006;103:16568-16573.

15. Riviere C, Richard T, Quentin L, Krisa S, Merillon JM, Monti JP. Inhibitory activity of stilbenes on Alzheimer's β-amyloid fibrils *in vitro*. *Bioorg Med Chem* 2007;15:1160-1167.

16. Penumathsa SV, Thirunavukkarasu M, Koneru S, Juhasz B, Zhan L, Pant R, Menon VP, Otani H, Maulik N. Statin and resveratrol in combination induces cardioprotection against myocardial infarction in hypercholesterolemic rat. *J Mol Cell Cardiol* 2006 (doi:10.1016/j.yjmcc.2006.10.018).

17. Penumathsa SV, Maulik N. Resveratrol: a promising agent in promoting cardioprotection against coronary heart disease. *Can J Physiol Pharmacol.* 2009;87(4):275-86.

18. El Bedoui J, Oak MH, Anglard P, Schini-Kerth VB. Catechins prevent vascular smooth muscle cell invasion by inhibiting MT1-MMP activity and MMP-2 expression. *Cardiovasc Res* 2005;67:317-325.

19. Wolfram S. Effects of green tea and EGCG on cardiovascular and metabolic health. *J Am Coll Nutr.* 2007;26(4):373S-388S.

20. McKay DL, Blumberg JB. Cranberries (Vaccinium macrocarpon) and cardiovascular disease risk factors. *Nutr Rev.* 2007;65(11):490-502.

21. Prior RL. Fruits and vegetables in the prevention of cellular oxidative damage. *Am J Clin Nutr* 2003;78:(Suppl.):570S-578S.

22. Moskaug JO, Carlsen H, Myhrstad MC, Blomhoff R. Polyphenols and glutathione synthesis regulation. *Am J Clin Nutr* 2005;81Suppl.):277S-283S.

23. Urpi-Sarda M, Zamora-Ros R, Lamuela-Raventos R, Cherubini A, Jauregui O, de la Torre R, Covas MI, Estruch R, Jaeger W, Andres-Lacueva C. HPLC-Tandem mass spectrometric method to characterize resveratrol metabolism in humans. *Clin Chem* 2007;53:292-299.

24. Carluccio MA, Siculella L, Ancora MA, Massaro M, Scoditti E, Storelli C, Visioli F, Distante A, De Caterina R. Olive oil and red wine antioxidant polyphenols inhibit endothelial activation: Antiatherogenic properties of Mediterranean diet phytochemicals. *Arterioscler Thromb Vasc Biol* 2003;23:622-629.

25. Thompson HJ, Heimendinger J, Diker A, O'Neill C, Haegele A, Meinecke B, Wolfe P, Sedlacek S, Zhu Z, Jiang W. Dietary botanical diversity affects the reduction of oxidative biomarkers in women due to high vegetable and fruit intake. *J Nutr* 2006;136:2207-2212.

Chapter 4

1. Eckstein F, Lemberger B, Gratzke C, Hudelmaier M, Glaser C, Englmeier KH, Reiser M. *In vivo* cartilage deformation after different types of activity and its dependence on physical training status. *Ann Rheum Dis* 2005;64:291-295.

2. Roos EM, Dahlberg L. Positive effects of moderate exercise on glycosaminoglycan content in knee cartilage: A four-month, randomized, controlled trial in patients at risk of osteoarthritis. *Arthritis Rheum* 2005;52:3507-3514.

3. Scott JE, Stockwell RA. Cartilage elasticity resides in shape module decoran and aggrecan sumps of damping fluid. Implications in osteoarthrosis. *J Physiol* 2006; Mar. 31. doi: 10.1113/jphysiol.2006.108100 (http://jp.physoc.org/cgi/content/abstract/jphysiol.2006.108100v1).

4. Modawal A, Ferrer M, Choi HK, Castle JA. Hyaluronic acid injections relieve knee pain. *J Fam Pract* 2005;54:758-767.

5. Aragona P, Papa V, Micali A, Santocono M, Milazzo G. Long term treatment with sodium hyaluronate-containing artificial tears reduces ocular surface damage in patients with dry eye. *Br J Ophthalmol* 2002;86:181-184.

6. Rotstein NP, Politi LE, German OL, Girotti R. Protective effect of docosahexaenoic acid on oxidative stress-induced apoptosis of retina photoreceptors. *Invest Ophthalmol Vis Sci* 2003;44:2252-2259.

7. Debbasch C, De La Salle SB, Brignole F, Rat P, Warnet JM, Baudouin C. Cytoprotective effects of hyaluronic acid and Carbomer 934P in ocular surface epithelial cells. *Invest Ophthalmol Vis Sci* 2002;43:3409-3415.

8. Guinot C, Malvy DJ, Ambroisine L, Latreille J, Mauger E, Tenenhaus M, Morizot F, Lopez S, Le Fur I, Tschachler E. Relative contribution of intrinsic vs extrinsic factors to skin aging as determined by a validated skin age score. *Arch Dermatol* 2002;138:1454-1460.

9. Toole BP. Hyaluronan is not just a goo! *J Clin Invest* 2000;106:335-336.

10. Trommer H, Neubert RH. Screening for new antioxidative compounds for topical administration using skin lipid model systems. *J Pharm Pharm Sci* 2005;8:494-506.

11. Sato T, Iwaso H. An Effectiveness Study of Hyaluronic Acid (Hyabest® (J)) in the Treatment of Osteoarthritis of the Knee. *J New Rem & Clin* 2008;57(2):128-137.

12. Balogh L, Polyak A, Mathe D, Kiraly R, Thuroczy J, Terez M, Janoki G, Ting Y, Bucci LR, Schauss AG. Absorption, uptake and tissue affinity of high-molecular-weight hyaluronan after oral administration in rats and dogs. *J Agric Food Chem* 2008 Nov 26;56(22):10582-93.

13. Ishibashi G, Yamagata T, Rikitake S, Takiguchi Y. Digestion and Fermentation of Hyaluronic Acid. *Journal for the Integrated Study of Dietary Habits* 2002; 13(2): 107-111.

Chapter 5

1. Grimm T, Skrabala R, Chovanova Z, Muchova J, Sumegova K, Liptakova A, Durackova Z, Hogger P. Single and multiple dose pharmacokinetics of maritime pine bark extract (Pycnogenol®)

after oral administration to healthy volunteers. *BMC Clin Pharmacol* 2006;6(1):4. doi:10.1186/1472-6904-6-4 (http://www.biomedcentral.com/1472-6904/6/4).

2. Schafer A, Chovanova Z, Muchova J, Sumegova K, Liptakova A, Durackova Z, Hogger P. Inhibition of COX-1 and COX-2 activity by plasma of human volunteers after ingestion of French maritime pine bark extract (Pycnogenol). *Biomed Pharmacother* 2006;60:5-9.

3. Dene BA, Maritim AC, Sanders RA, Watkins JB 3rd. Effects of antioxidant treatment on normal and diabetic rat retinal enzyme activities. *J Ocul Pharmacol Ther* 2005;21:28-35.

4. Belcaro G, Cesarone MR, Errichi BM, Ledda A, Di Renzo A, Stuard S, Dugall M, Pellegrini L, Rohdewald P, Ippolito E, Ricci A, Cacchio M, Ruffini I, Fano F, Hosoi M. Venous ulcers: Microcirculatory improvement and faster healing with local use of Pycnogenol. *Angiology* 2005;56:699-705.

5. Cesarone MR, Belcaro G, Rohdewald P, Pellegrini L, Ledda A, Vinciguerra G, Ricci A, Gizzi G, Ippolito E, Fano F, Dugall M, Acerbi G, Cacchio M, Di Renzo A, Hosoi M, Stuard S, Corsi M. Comparison of Pycnogenol and Daflon in treating chronic venous insufficiency: A prospective, controlled study. *Clin Appl Thromb Hemost* 2006;12:205-212.

6. G. Belcaro, M. R. Cesarone, B. M. Errichi, A. Ledda, A. Di Renzo, S. Stuard, M. Dugall, L. Pellegrini, G. Gizzi, P. Rohdewald, E. Ippolito, A. Ricci, M. Cacchio, G. Cipollone, I. Ruffini, F. Fano, M. Hosoi. Diabetic ulcers: Microcirculatory improvement and faster healing with Pycnogenol. *Clin Appl Thromb Hem* 2006;12:318-323.

7. Vinciguerra G, Belcaro G, Cesarone MR, Rohdewald P, Stuard S, Ricci A, Di Renzo A, Hosoi M, Dugall M, Ledda A, Cacchio M, Acerbi G, Fano F. Cramps and muscular pain: Prevention with pycnogenol in normal subjects, venous patients, athletes, claudicants and in diabetic microangiopathy. *Angiology* 2006;57:331-339.

8. Cesarone MR, Belcaro G, Rohdewald P, Pellegrini L, Ippolito E, Scoccianti M, Ricci A, Dugall M, Cacchio M, Ruffini I, Fano F, Acerbi G, Vinciguerra MG, Bavera P, Di Renzo A, Errichi BM, Mucci F. Prevention of edema in long flights with Pycnogenol. *Clin Appl Thromb Hemost* 2005;11:289-294.

9. Trebatická J, Kopasová S, Hradecná Z, Cinovský K, Skodácek I, Suba J, Muchová J, Zitnanová I, Waczulíková I, Rohdewald P, Duracková Z. Treatment of ADHD with French maritime pine bark extract, Pycnogenol. *Eur Child Adolesc Psychiatry*. 2006;15(6):329-35.

10. Dvoráková M, Sivonová M, Trebatická J, Skodácek I, Waczuliková I, Muchová J, Duracková Z. The effect of polyphenolic extract from pine bark, Pycnogenol on the level of glutathione in children suffering from attention deficit hyperactivity disorder (ADHD).*Redox Rep.* 2006;11(4):163-72.

11. Ryan J, Croft K, Mori T, Wesnes K, Spong J, Downey L, Kure C, Lloyd J, Stough C. An examination of the effects of the antioxidant Pycnogenol on cognitive performance, serum lipid profile,

endocrinological and oxidative stress biomarkers in an elderly population. *J Psychopharmacol.* 2008;22(5):553-62.

Chapter 6

1. Henning SM, Niu Y, Lee NH, Thames GD, Minutti RR, Wang H, Go VL, Heber D. Bioavailability and antioxidant activity of tea flavanols after consumption of green tea, black tea, or a green tea extract supplement. *Am J Clin Nutr* 2004;80:1558-1564.
2. Seeram NP, Henning SM, Niu Y, Lee R, Scheuller HS, Heber D. Catechin and caffeine content of green tea dietary supplements and correlation with antioxidant capacity. *J Agric Food Chem* 2006;54:1599-1603.
3. Leung LK, Su Y, Chen R, Zhang Z, Huang Y, Chen ZY. Theaflavins in black tea and catechins in green tea are equally effective antioxidants. *J Nutr* 2001;131:2248-2251.
4. Vinson JA, Dabbagh YA. Effect of green and black tea supplementation on lipids, lipid oxidation and fibrinogen in the hamster: Mechanisms for the epidemiological benefits of tea drinking. *FEBS Lett* 1998;433:44-46.
5. Hakim IA, Harris RB, Brown S, Chow HH, Wiseman S, Agarwal S, Talbot W. Effect of increased tea consumption on oxidative DNA damage among smokers: A randomized controlled study. *J Nutr* 2003;133:3303S-3309S.
6. Hakim IA, Harris RB, Chow HH, Dean M, Brown S, Ali IU. Effect of a 4-month tea intervention on oxidative DNA damage among heavy smokers: Role of glutathione S-transferase genotypes. *Cancer Epidemiol Biomarkers Prev* 2004;13:242-249.
7. Food and Drug Administration. Department of Health and Human Services. Final Rule Declaring Dietary Supplements Containing Ephedrine Alkaloids Adulterated Because They Present an Unreasonable Risk; Final Rule. *Fed Reg* 2004;69:6787-6854.
8. Winkelmayer WC, Stampfer MJ, Willett WC, Curhan GC. Habitual caffeine intake and the risk of hypertension in women. *JAMA* 2005;294:2330-2335.
9. Yang YC, Lu FH, Wu JS, Wu CH, Chang CJ. The protective effect of habitual tea consumption on hypertension. *Arch Intern Med* 2004;164:1534-1540.
10. Hodgson JM, Devine A, Puddey IB, Chan SY, Beilin LJ, Prince RL. Tea intake is inversely related to blood pressure in older women. *J Nutr* 2003;133:2883-2886.
11. Sano J, Inami S, Seimiya K, Ohba T, Sakai S, Takano T, Mizuno K. Effects of green tea intake on the development of coronary artery disease. *Circ J* 2004;68:665-670.
12. Arts IC, Hollman PC, Feskens EJ, Bueno de Mesquita HB, Kromhout D. Catechin intake might explain the inverse relation between tea consumption and ischemic heart disease: The Zutphen Elderly Study. *Am J Clin Nutr* 2001;74:227-232.

13. Peters U, Poole C, Arab L. Does tea affect cardiovascular disease? A meta-analysis. *Am J Epidemiol* 2001;154:495-503.
14. Mukamal KJ, Maclure M, Muller JE, Sherwood JB, Mittleman MA. Tea consumption and mortality after acute myocardial infarction. *Circulation* 2002;105:2476-2481.
15. El Bedoui J, Oak MH, Anglard P, Schini-Kerth VB. Catechins prevent vascular smooth muscle cell invasion by inhibiting MT1-MMP activity and MMP-2 expression. *Cardiovasc Res* 2005;67:317-325.
16. Ilich JZ, Brownbill RA, Tamborini L, Crncevic-Orlic Z. To drink or not to drink: How are alcohol, caffeine and past smoking related to bone mineral density in elderly women? *J Am Coll Nutr* 2002;21:536-544.
17. Kiel DP, Felson DT, Hannan MT, Anderson JJ, Wilson PW. Caffeine and the risk of hip fracture: The Framingham Study. *Am J Epidemiol* 1990;132:675-684.
18. Rapuri PB, Gallagher JC, Kinyamu HK, Ryschon KL. Caffeine intake increases the rate of bone loss in elderly women and interacts with vitamin D receptor genotypes. *Am J Clin Nutr* 2001;74:694-700.
19. Lloyd T, Rollings NJ, Kieselhorst K, Eggli DF, Mauger E. Dietary caffeine intake is not correlated with adolescent bone gain. *J Am Coll Nutr* 1998;17:454-457.
20. Lloyd T, Johnson-Rollings N, Eggli DF, Kieselhorst K, Mauger EA, Cusatis DC. Bone status among postmenopausal women with different habitual caffeine intakes: A longitudinal investigation. *J Am Coll Nutr* 2000;19:256-261.
21. Chen Z, Pettinger MB, Ritenbaugh C, LaCroix AZ, Robbins J, Caan BJ, Barad DH, Hakim IA. Habitual tea consumption and risk of osteoporosis: A prospective study in the Women's Health Initiative Observational Cohort. *Am J Epidemiol* 2003;158:772-781.
22. Wu CH, Lu FH, Chang CS, Chang TC, Wang RH, Chang CJ. Relationship among habitual tea consumption, percent body fat, and body fat distribution. *Obes Res* 2003;11:1088-1095.
23. Wolfram S, Wang Y, Thielecke F. Anti-obesity effects of green tea: From bedside to bench. *Mol Nutr Food Res* 2006;50:176-187.
24. Murase T, Haramizu S, Shimotoyodome A, Tokimitsu I, Hase T. Green tea extract improves running endurance in mice by stimulating lipid utilization during exercise. *Am J Physiol Regul Integr Comp Physiol* 2006;290:R1550-R1556.
25. Dulloo AG, Duret C, Rohrer D, Girardier L, Mensi N, Fathi M, Chantre P, Vandermander J. Efficacy of a green tea extract rich in catechin polyphenols and caffeine in increasing 24-h energy expenditure and fat oxidation in humans. *Am J Clin Nutr* 1999;70:1040-1045.
26. Chantre P, Lairon D. Recent findings of green tea extract AR25 (Exolise) and its activity for the treatment of obesity. *Phytomedicine* 2002;9:3-8.
27. Nagao T, Komine Y, Soga S, Meguro S, Hase T, Tanaka Y, Tokimitsu I. Ingestion of a tea rich in catechins leads to a reduction in body fat and malondialdehyde-modified LDL in men. *Am J Clin Nutr*

2005;81:122-129.
28.   Rosmond R, Dallman MF, Bjorntorp P. Stress-related cortisol
       secretion in men: Relationships with abdominal obesity and
       endocrine, metabolic and hemodynamic abnormalities. *J Clin
       Endocrinol Metab* 1998;83:1853-1859.
29.   Juneja LR, Chu D-C, Okubo T, Nagato Y, Yokogoshi H. L-theanine, a
       unique amino acid of green tea and its relaxation effect in humans.
       Trends Food Sci Technol 1999;10:199-204.
30.   Zheng G, Sayama K, Okubo T, Juneja LR, Oguni I. Anti-obesity effects
       of three major components of green tea, catechins, caffeine and
       theanine, in mice. *In Vivo* 2004;18:55-62.
31.   Curhan GC, Willett WC, Speizer FE, Stampfer MJ. Beverage use and
       risk of kidney stones in women. *Ann Intern Med* 1998;128:534-540.
32.   Curhan GC, Willett WC, Rimm EB, Spiegelman D, Stampfer MJ.
       Prospective study of beverage use and the risk of kidney stones. *Am J
       Epidemiol* 1996;143:240-247.
33.   Yu, H., Oho, T., Xu, L. X. Effects of several tea components on acid
       resistance of human tooth enamel. *J Dent* 1995;13:101-105.
34.   Linke HA, LeGeros RZ. Black tea extract and dental caries formation
       in hamsters. *Int J Food Sci Nutr* 2003;54:89-95.
35.   Lorenz M, Urban J, Engelhardt U, Baumann G, Stangl K, Stangl V.
       Green and black tea are equally potent stimuli of NO production
       and vasodilation: new insights into tea ingredients involved. *Basic
       Res Cardiol* 2009;104(1):100-10.
36.   Lin CL, Huang HC, Lin JK. Theaflavins attenuate hepatic lipid
       accumulation through activating AMPK in human HepG2 cells. *J
       Lipid Res* 2007;48(11):2334-43.
37.   Maron DJ, Lu GP, Cai NS, Wu ZG, Li YH, Chen H, Zhu JQ, Jin XJ,
       Wouters BC, Zhao J. Cholesterol-lowering effect of a theaflavin-
       enriched green tea extract: a randomized controlled trial. *Arch Intern
       Med* 2003;163(12):1448-53.

Chapter 7

1.   Brufau G, Canela MA, Rafecas M. Phytosterols: physiologic and
       metabolic aspects related to cholesterol-lowering properties. Nutr
       Res. 2008 Apr;28(4):217-25.
2.   Food and Drug Administration. Food Labeling: Health Claims; Plant
       Sterol/Stanol Esters and Coronary Heart Disease; Interim Final Rule.
       Fed Reg 2000;65:54685-54739.
3.   Quilez J, Rafecas M, Brufau G, Garcia-Lorda P, Megias I, Bullo
       M, Ruiz JA, Salas-Salvado J. Bakery products enriched with
       phytosterol esters, -tocopherol and -carotene decrease plasma
       LDL-cholesterol and maintain plasma -carotene concentrations in
       normocholesterolemic men and women. *J Nutr* 2003;133:3103-3109.
4.   Vanstone CA, Raeini-Sarjaz M, Parsons WE, Jones PJ. Unesterified
       plant sterols and stanols lower LDL-cholesterol concentrations
       equivalently in hypercholesterolemic persons. *Am J Clin Nutr*

2002;76:1272-1278.
5. Brufau G, Canela MA, Rafecas M. Phytosterols: physiologic and metabolic aspects related to cholesterol-lowering properties. Nutr Res. 2008 Apr;28(4):217-25.
6. Demonty I, Ras RT, van der Knaap HC, Duchateau GS, Meijer L, Zock PL, Geleijnse JM, Trautwein EA.Continuous dose-response relationship of the LDL-cholesterol-lowering effect of phytosterol intake. J Nutr. 2009 Feb;139(2):271-84.

Chapter 8

1. Rahman K, Lowe GM. Garlic and cardiovascular disease: A critical review. *J Nutr* 2006;136(Suppl.):736S-740S.
2. Weiss N, Ide N, Abahji T, Nill L, Keller C, Hoffmann U. Aged garlic extract improves homocysteine-induced endothelial dysfunction in macro- and microcirculation. *J Nutr* 2006;136(Suppl.):750S-754S.
3. Lau BH. Suppression of LDL oxidation by garlic compounds is a possible mechanism of cardiovascular health benefit. *J Nutr* 2006;136(Suppl.):765S-768S.
4. Ide N, Keller C, Weiss N. Aged garlic extract inhibits homocysteine-induced CD36 expression and foam cell formation in human macrophages. *J Nutr* 2006;136(Suppl.):755S-758S.
5. Ahmad MS, Ahmed N. Antiglycation properties of aged garlic extract: Possible role in prevention of diabetic complications. *J Nutr* 2006;136(Suppl.):796S-799S.
6. Gonen A, Harats D, Rabinkov A, Miron T, Mirelman D, Wilchek M, Weiner L, Ulman E, Levkovitz H, Ben-Shushan D, Shaish A. The antiatherogenic effect of allicin: Possible mode of action. *Pathobiology* 2005;72:325-334.
7. Singh DK, Porter TD. Inhibition of sterol 4 -methyl oxidase is the principal mechanism by which garlic decreases cholesterol synthesis. *J Nutr* 2006;136(Suppl.):759S-764S.
8. Ried K, Frank OR, Stocks NP, Fakler P, Sullivan T. Effect of garlic on blood pressure: a systematic review and meta-analysis. *BMC Cardiovasc Disord* 2008;8:13.
9. Reinhart KM, Coleman CI, Teevan C, Vachhani P, White CM. Effects of garlic on blood pressure in patients with and without systolic hypertension: a meta-analysis. *Ann Pharmacother* 2008;42(12):1766-71.
10. Morihara N, Nishihama T, Ushijima M, Ide N, Takeda H, Hayama M. Garlic as an anti-fatigue agent.*Mol Nutr Food Res* 2007;51(11):1329-34.
11. Patya M, Zahalka MA, Vanichkin A, Rabinkov A, Miron T, Mirelman D, Wilchek M, Lander HM, Novogrodsky A. Allicin stimulates lymphocytes and elicits an antitumor effect: A possible role of p21[ras]. *Int Immunol* 2004;16:275-281.
12.. Zhang ZM, Zhong N, Gao HQ, Zhang SZ, Wei Y, Xin H, Mei X, Hou HS, Lin XY, Shi Q. Inducing apoptosis and upregulation of Bax and

Fas ligand expression by allicin in hepatocellular carcinoma in Balb/c nude mice. *Chin Med J* 2006;119:422-425.

Chapter 9

1. Lenaz G, Parenti Castelli G, Fato, D'Aurelio M, Bovina C, Formiggini G, Marchetti M, Estornell E, Rauchova H. Coenzyme Q deficiency in mitochondria: Kinetic saturation versus physical saturation. *Mol Aspects Med* 1997;18 (Suppl.):S25-S31.
2. Sander S, Coleman CI, Patel AA, Kluger J, White CM. The impact of coenzyme Q_{10} on systolic function in patients with chronic heart failure. *J Card Fail* 2006;12:464-472.
3. Belardinelli R, Mucaj A, Lacalaprice F, Solenghi M, Seddaiu G, Principi F, Tiano L, Littarru GP. Coenzyme Q_{10} and exercise training in chronic heart failure. *Eur Heart J* 2006; Aug 1.
4. Lalani SR, Vladutiu GD, Plunkett K, Lotze TE, Adesina AM, Scaglia F. Isolated mitochondrial myopathy associated with muscle coenzyme Q_{10} deficiency. *Arch Neurol* 2005;62:317-320.
5. Di Lisa F, Menabo R, Canton M, Barile M, Bernardi P. Opening of the mitochondrial permeability transition pore causes depletion of mitochondrial and cytosolic NAD^+ and is a causative event in the death of myocytes in postischemic reperfusion of the heart. *J Biol Chem* 2001;276:2571-2575.
6. Ochoa JJ, Quiles JL, Huertas JR, Mataix J. Coenzyme Q_{10} protects from aging-related oxidative stress and improves mitochondrial function in heart of rats fed a polyunsaturated fatty acid (PUFA)-rich diet. *J Gerontol A Biol Sci Med Sci* 2005;60:970-975.
7. Somayajulu M, McCarthy S, Hung M, Sikorska M, Borowy-Borowski H, Pandey S. Role of mitochondria in neuronal cell death induced by oxidative stress; neuroprotection by Coenzyme Q10. *Neurobiol Dis* 2005;18:618-627.
8. Huertas JR, Martinez-Velasco E, Ibanez S, Lopez-Frias M, Ochoa JJ, Quiles J, Parenti Castelli G, Mataix J, Lenaz G. Virgin olive oil and coenzyme Q_{10} protect heart mitochondria from peroxidative damage during aging. *Biofactors* 1999;9:337-343.
9. enova ML, Pich MM, Biondi A, Bernacchia A, Falasca A, Bovina C, Formiggini G, Parenti Castelli G, Lenaz G. Mitochondrial production of oxygen radical species and the role of Coenzyme Q as an antioxidant. *Exp Biol Med* 2003;228:506-513.
10. Fernandez-Ayala DJ, Lopez-Lluch G, Garcia-Valdes M, Arroyo A, Navas P. Specificity of coenzyme Q_{10} for a balanced function of respiratory chain and endogenous ubiquinone biosynthesis in human cells. *Biochim Biophys Acta* 2005;1706:174-183.
11. Arroyo A, Navarro F, Gomez-Diaz C, Crane FL, Alcain FJ, Navas P, Villalba JM. Interactions between ascorbyl free radical and coenzyme Q at the plasma membrane. *J Bioenerg Biomembr* 2000;32:199-210.
12. Lass A, Sohal RS. Effect of coenzyme Q(10) and alpha-tocopherol content of mitochondria on the production of superoxide anion

radicals. *FASEB J* 2000;14:87-94.

13. Mabuchi H, Higashikata T, Kawashiri M, Katsuda S, Mizuno M, Nohara A, Inazu A, Koizumi J, Kobayashi J. Reduction of serum ubiquinol-10 and ubiquinone-10 levels by atorvastatin in hypercholesterolemic patients. *J Atheroscler Thromb* 2005;12:111-119.

14. Rundek T, Naini A, Sacco R, Coates K, DiMauro S. Atorvastatin decreases the coenzyme Q10 level in the blood of patients at risk for cardiovascular disease and stroke. *Arch Neurol* 2004;61:889-892.

15. Thompson PD, Clarkson P, Karas RH. Statin-associated myopathy. *JAMA* 2003;289:1681-1690.

16. Tomlinson SS, Mangione KK. Potential adverse effects of statins on muscle. *Phys Ther* 2005;85:459-465.

17. Baker SK. Molecular clues into the pathogenesis of statin-mediated muscle toxicity. *Muscle Nerve* 2005;31:572-580.

18. Paiva H, Thelen KM, Van Coster R, Smet J, De Paepe B, Mattila KM, Laakso J, Lehtimaki T, von Bergmann K, Lutjohann D, Laaksonen R. High-dose statins and skeletal muscle metabolism in humans: A randomized, controlled trial. *Clin Pharmacol Ther* 2005;78:60-68.

19. Baker SK, Tarnopolsky MA. Statin-associated neuromyotoxicity. *Drugs Today* 2005;41:267-293.

20. Nawarskas JJ. HMG-CoA reductase inhibitors and coenzyme Q_{10}. *Cardiol Rev* 2005;13:76-79.

21. Ferrante KL, Shefner J, Zhang H, Betensky R, O'Brien M, Yu H, Fantasia M, Taft J, Beal MF, Traynor B, Newhall K, Donofrio P, Caress J, Ashburn C, Freiberg B, O'Neill C, Paladenech C, Walker T, Pestronk A, Abrams B, Florence J, Renna R, Schierbecker J, Malkus B, Cudkowicz M. Tolerance of high-dose (3,000 mg/day) coenzyme Q_{10} in ALS. *Neurology* 2005;65:1834-1836.

22. Chopra RK, Goldman R, Sinatra ST, Bhagavan HN. Relative bioavailability of coenzyme Q10 formulations in human subjects. *Intern J Vit Nutr Res* 1998;68:109-113.

Chapter 10

1. Ray AL, Semba RD, Walston J, Ferrucci L, Cappola AR, Ricks MO, Xue QL, Fried LP. Low serum selenium and total carotenoids predict mortality among older women living in the community: The Women's Health and Aging Studies. *J Nutr* 2006;136:172-176.

2. Durga J, van Boxtel MP, Schouten EG, Kok FJ, Jolles J, Katan MB, Verhoef P. Effect of 3-year folic acid supplementation on cognitive function in older adults in the FACIT trial: A randomised, double blind, controlled trial. *Lancet* 2007;369:208-216.

3. Durga J, Verhoef P, Anteunis LJ, Schouten E, Kok FJ. Effects of folic acid supplementation on hearing in older adults: A randomized, controlled trial. *Ann Intern Med* 2007;146:1-9.

4. McCracken C, Hudson P, Ellis R, McCaddon A; Medical Research Council Cognitive Function and Ageing Study. Methylmalonic acid and cognitive function in the Medical Research Council Cognitive

Function and Ageing Study. *Am J Clin Nutr* 2006;84:1406-1411.
5.   Feng L, Ng TP, Chuah L, Niti M, Kua EH. Homocysteine, folate, and vitamin B-12 and cognitive performance in older Chinese adults: Findings from the Singapore Longitudinal Ageing Study. *Am J Clin Nutr* 2006;84:1506-1512.
6.   Tucker KL, Qiao N, Scott T, Rosenberg I, Spiro A. High homocysteine and low B vitamins predict cognitive decline in aging men: The Veterans Affairs Normative Aging Study. *Am J Clin Nutr* 2005;82:627-635.
7.   Mooijaart SP, Gussekloo J, Frolich M, Jolles J, Stott DJ, Westendorp RG, de Craen AJ. Homocysteine, vitamin B-12, and folic acid and the risk of cognitive decline in old age: The Leiden 85-Plus study. *Am J Clin Nutr* 2005;82:866-871.
8.   Duthie SJ, Whalley LJ, Collins AR, Leaper S, Berger K, Deary IJ. Homocysteine, B vitamin status, and cognitive function in the elderly. *Am J Clin Nutr* 2002;75:908-913.
9.   Ravaglia G, Forti P, Maioli F, Martelli M, Servadei L, Brunetti N, Porcellini E, Licastro F. Homocysteine and folate as risk factors for dementia and Alzheimer disease. *Am J Clin Nutr* 2005;82:636-643.
10. Oliveira FA, Galan DT, Ribeiro AM, Santos Cruz J. Thiamine deficiency during pregnancy leads to cerebellar neuronal death in rat offspring: Role of voltage-dependent K(+) channels. *Brain Res* 2007;1134:79-86.
11. Dai X, Sun Y, Jiang Z. Protective effects of vitamin E against oxidative damage induced by Aβ(1-40)Cu(II) complexes. *Acta Biochim Biophys Sin* 2007;39:123-130.
12. Hill KE, Zhou J, Austin LM, Motley AK, Ham AJ, Olson GE, Atkins JF, Gesteland RF, Burk RF. The selenium-rich C-terminal domain of mouse selenoprotein P is necessary for supply of selenium to brain and testis but not for maintenance of whole-body selenium. *J Biol Chem* 2007 Feb 20 (www.jbc.org/cgi/doi/10.1074/jbc.M700436200).
13. Manju L, Nair RR. Magnesium deficiency augments myocardial response to reactive oxygen species. *Can J Physiol Pharmacol* 2006;84:617-624.
14. Song Y, Ridker PM, Manson JE, Cook NR, Buring JE, Liu S. Magnesium intake, C-reactive protein, and the prevalence of metabolic syndrome in middle-aged and older U.S. women. *Diabetes Care* 2005;28:1438-1444.
15. He K, Liu K, Daviglus ML, Morris SJ, Loria CM, Van Horn L, Jacobs DR Jr, Savage PJ. Magnesium intake and incidence of metabolic syndrome among young adults. *Circulation* 2006;113:1675-1682.
16. Kousa A, Havulinna AS, Moltchanova E, Taskinen O, Nikkarinen M, Eriksson J, Karvonen M. Calcium:magnesium ratio in local groundwater and incidence of acute myocardial infarction among males in rural Finland. *Environ Health Perspect* 2006;114:730-734.
17. Heaney RP. Calcium intake and disease prevention. *Arq Bras Endocrinol Metabol* 2006;50:685-693.
18. Jackson RD, LaCroix AZ, Gass M, Wallace RB, Robbins J, Lewis CE,

Bassford T, Beresford SA, Black HR, Blanchette P, Bonds DE, Brunner RL, Brzyski RG, Caan B, Cauley JA, Chlebowski RT, Cummings SR, Granek I, Hays J, Heiss G, Hendrix SL, Howard BV, Hsia J, Hubbell FA, Johnson KC, Judd H, Kotchen JM, Kuller LH, Langer RD, Lasser NL, Limacher MC, Ludlam S, Manson JE, Margolis KL, McGowan J, Ockene JK, O'Sullivan MJ, Phillips L, Prentice RL, Sarto GE, Stefanick ML, Van Horn L, Wactawski-Wende J, Whitlock E, Anderson GL, Assaf AR, Barad D; Women's Health Initiative Investigators. Calcium plus vitamin D supplementation and the risk of fractures. *N Engl J Med* 2006;354:669-683.

19. Bischoff-Ferrari HA, Willett WC, Wong JB, Giovannucci E, Dietrich T, Dawson-Hughes B. Fracture prevention with vitamin D supplementation: A meta-analysis of randomized controlled trials. *JAMA* 2005;293:2257-2264.

20. Ryder KM, Shorr RI, Bush AJ, Kritchevsky SB, Harris T, Stone K, Cauley J, Tylavsky FA. Magnesium intake from food and supplements is associated with bone mineral density in healthy older white subjects. *J Am Geriatr Soc* 2005;53:1875-1880.

21. Carpenter TO, DeLucia MC, Zhang JH, Bejnerowicz G, Tartamella L, Dziura J, Petersen KF, Befroy D, Cohen D. A randomized controlled study of effects of dietary magnesium oxide supplementation on bone mineral content in healthy girls. *J Clin Endocrinol Metab* 2006;91:4866-4872.

22. Macdonald HM, New SA, Golden MH, Campbell MK, Reid DM. Nutritional associations with bone loss during the menopausal transition: Evidence of a beneficial effect of calcium, alcohol, and fruit and vegetable nutrients and of a detrimental effect of fatty acids. *Am J Clin Nutr* 2004;79:155-165.

23. Cerhan JR, Saag KG, Merlino LA, Mikuls TR, Criswell LA. Antioxidant micronutrients and risk of rheumatoid arthritis in a cohort of older women. *Am J Epidemiol* 2003;157:345-354.

24. McAlindon TE, Jacques P, Zhang Y, Hannan MT, Aliabadi P, Weissman B, Rush D, Levy D, Felson DT. Do antioxidant micronutrients protect against the development and progression of knee osteoarthritis? *Arthritis Rheum* 1996;39:648-656.

25. Surapaneni KM, Venkataramana G. Status of lipid peroxidation, glutathione, ascorbic acid, vitamin E and antioxidant enzymes in patients with osteoarthritis. *Indian J Med Sci* 2007;61:9-14.

26. Devirian TA, Volpe SL. The physiological effects of dietary boron. *Crit Rev Food Sci Nutr.* 2003;43(2):219-31.

27. Cockayne S, Adamson J, Lanham-New S, Shearer MJ, Gilbody S, Torgerson DJ. Vitamin K and the prevention of fractures: Systematic review and meta-analysis of randomized controlled trials. *Arch Intern Med* 2006;166:1256-1261.

28. Etminan M, FitzGerald JM, Gleave M, Chambers K. Intake of selenium in the prevention of prostate cancer: A systematic review and meta-analysis. *Cancer Causes Control* 2005;16:1125-1131.

29. Sabichi AL, Lee JJ, Taylor RJ, Thompson IM, Miles BJ, Tangen CM,

Minasian LM, Pisters LL, Caton JR, Basler JW, Lerner SP, Menter DG, Marshall JR, Crawford ED, Lippman SM. Selenium accumulation in prostate tissue during a randomized, controlled short-term trial of L-selenomethionine: A Southwest Oncology Group Study. *Clin Cancer Res* 2006;12:2178-2184.

30. Weinstein SJ, Wright ME, Pietinen P, King I, Tan C, Taylor PR, Virtamo J, Albanes D. Serum α-tocopherol and γ-tocopherol in relation to prostate cancer risk in a prospective study. *J Natl Cancer Inst* 2005;97:396-399.

31. Kirsh VA, Hayes RB, Mayne ST, Chatterjee N, Subar AF, Dixon LB, Albanes D, Andriole GL, Urban DA, Peters U; PLCO Trial. Supplemental and dietary vitamin E, beta-carotene, and vitamin C intakes and prostate cancer risk. *J Natl Cancer Inst* 2006;98:245-254.

32. Costello LC, Franklin RB. The clinical relevance of the metabolism of prostate cancer; zinc and tumor suppression: Connecting the dots. *Mol Cancer* 2006;5:17 (13 pages). doi:10.1186/1476-4598-5-17 (http://www.molecular-cancer.com/content/5/1/17).

33. Huerta MG, Roemmich JN, Kington ML, Bovbjerg VE, Weltman AL, Holmes VF, Patrie JT, Rogol AD, Nadler JL. Magnesium deficiency is associated with insulin resistance in obese children. *Diabetes Care* 2005;28:1175-1181.

34. Song Y, Ridker PM, Manson JE, Cook NR, Buring JE, Liu S. Magnesium intake, C-reactive protein, and the prevalence of metabolic syndrome in middle-aged and older U.S. women. *Diabetes Care* 2005;28:1438-1444.

35. Lopez-Ridaura R, Willett WC, Rimm EB, Liu S, Stampfer MJ, Manson JE, Hu FB. Magnesium intake and risk of type 2 diabetes in men and women. *Diabetes Care* 2004;27:134-140.

36. Schauber J, Dorschner RA, Coda AB, Buchau AS, Liu PT, Kiken D, Helfrich YR, Kang S, Elalieh HZ, Steinmeyer A, Zugel U, Bikle DD, Modlin RL, Gallo RL. Injury enhances TLR2 function and antimicrobial peptide expression through a vitamin D-dependent mechanism. *J Clin Invest* 2007;117:803-811.

37. Simasek M, Blandino DA Treatment of the common cold. *Am Fam Physician* 2007;75:515-520.

38. Stromberg SP, Carlson J. Robustness and fragility in immunosenescence. *PLoS Comput Biol* 2006;2:e160 (doi:10.1371/journal.pcbi.0020160).

39. Broome CS, McArdle F, Kyle JAM, Andrews F, Lowe NM, Hart CA, Arthur JR, Jackson MJ. An increase in selenium intake imprioves immune function and poliovirus handling in adults with marginal selenium statrus. *Am J Clin Nutr* 2004;80:154-162.

40. Depeint F, Bruce WR, Shangari N, Mehta R, O'Brien PJ. Mitochondrial function and toxicity: Role of the B vitamin family on mitochondrial energy metabolism. *Chem Biol Interact* 2006;163:94-112.

41. Meisel P, Schwahn C, Luedemann J, John U, Kroemer HK, Kocher T. Magnesium deficiency is associated with periodontal disease. *J Dent*

Res 2005;84:937-941.

Chapter 11

1. Serra-Majem L, Roman B, Estruch R. Scientific evidence of interventions using the Mediterranean diet: A systematic review. *Nutr Rev* 2006;64:S27-S47.
2. Colomer R, Menendez JA. Mediterranean diet, olive oil and cancer. *Clin Transl Oncol* 2006;8:15-21.
3. Simopoulos AP. The Mediterranean diets: What is so special about the diet of Greece? The scientific evidence. *J Nutr* 2001;131:3065S-3073S.
4. Trichopoulou A, Lagiou P, Kuper H, Trichopoulos D. Cancer and Mediterranean dietary traditions. *Cancer Epidemiol Biomarkers Prev* 2000;9:869-873.
5. La Vecchia C. Mediterranean diet and cancer. *Public Health Nutr* 2004;7:965-968.
6. Estruch R, Martinez-Gonzalez MA, Corella D, Salas-Salvado J, Ruiz-Gutierrez V, Covas MI, Fiol M, Gomez-Gracia E, Lopez-Sabater MC, Vinyoles E, Aros F, Conde M, Lahoz C, Lapetra J, Saez G, Ros E; PREDIMED Study Investigators. Effects of a Mediterranean-style diet on cardiovascular risk factors: A randomized trial. *Ann Intern Med* 2006;145:1-11.
7. Schroder H, Marrugat J, Vila J, Covas MI, Elosua R. Adherence to the traditional Mediterranean diet is inversely associated with body mass index and obesity in a Spanish population. *J Nutr* 2004;134:3355-3361.
8. Covas MI, Nyyssonen K, Poulsen HE, Kaikkonen J, Zunft HJ, Kiesewetter H, Gaddi A, de la Torre R, Mursu J, Baumler H, Nascetti S, Salonen JT, Fito M, Virtanen J, Marrugat J, EUROLIVE Study Group. The effect of polyphenols in olive oil on heart disease risk factors: A randomized trial. *Ann Intern Med* 2006;145:333-341.
9. Carluccio MA, Siculella L, Ancora MA, Massaro M, Scoditti E, Storelli C, Visioli F, Distante A, De Caterina R. Olive oil and red wine antioxidant polyphenols inhibit endothelial activation: Antiatherogenic properties of Mediterranean diet phytochemicals. *Arterioscler Thromb Vasc Biol* 2003;23:622-629.
10. Fernandez-Jarne E, Martinez-Losa E, Prado-Santamaria M, Brugarolas-Brufau C, Serrano-Martinez M, Martinez-Gonzalez MA. Risk of first non-fatal myocardial infarction negatively associated with olive oil consumption: A case-control study in Spain. *Intern J Epidemiol* 2002;31:474-480.
11. Pechanova O, Rezzani R, Babal P, Bernatova I, Andriantsitohaina R. Beneficial effects of provinols: Cardiovascular system and kidney. *Physiol Res* 2006;55(Suppl. 1):S17-S30.
12. Puzserova A, Csizmadiova Z, Andriantsitohaina R, Bernatova I. Vascular effects of red wine polyphenols in chronic stress-exposed Wistar-Kyoto rats. *Physiol Res* 2006;55(Suppl. 1):S39-S47.

13.   Szmitko PE, Verma S. Antiatherogenic potential of red wine: Clinician update. *Am J Physiol Heart Circ Physiol* 2005;288:H2023-H2030.

Chapter 12

1.   Lee I-M, Paffenbarger RS Jr. Associations of light, moderate, and vigorous intensity physical activity with longevity. The Harvard Alumni Health Study. *Am J Epidemiol* 2000;151:293-299.
2.   Katzmarzyk PT, Church TS, Blair SN. Cardiorespiratory fitness attenuates the effects of the metabolic syndrome on all-cause and cardiovascular disease mortality in men. *Arch Intern Med* 2004;164:1092-1097.
3.   Hu FB, Willett WC, Li T, Stampfer MJ, Colditz GA, Manson JAE. Adiposity as compared with physical activity in predicting mortality among women. *N Engl J Med* 2004;351:2694-2703.
4.   Iestra JA, Kromhout D, van der Schouw YT, Grobbee DE, Boshuizen HC, van Staveren WA. Effect size estimates of lifestyle and dietary changes on all-cause mortality in coronary disease patients. A systematic review. *Circulation* 2005;112:924-934.
5.   Oguma Y, Sesso HD, Paffenbarger RS Jr, Lee I-M. Physical activity and all cause mortality in women: A review of the evidence. *Br J Sports Med* 2002;36:162-172.
6.   Whang W, Manson JAE, Hu FB, Chae CU, Rexrode KM, Willett WC, Stampfer MJ, Albert CM. Physical exertion, exercise, and sudden cardiac death in women. *JAMA* 2006;295:1399-1403.
7.   Albert CM, Mittleman MA, Chae CU, Lee IM, Hennekens CH, Manson JE. Triggering of sudden death from cardiac causes by vigorous exertion. *N Engl J Med* 2000;343:1355-1361.
8.   Tanasescu M, Leitzmann MF, Rimm EB, Willett WC, Stampfer MJ, Hu FB. Exercise type and intensity in relation to coronary heart disease in men. *JAMA* 2002;288:1994-2000.
9.   Manson JE, Greenland P, LaCroix AZ, Stefanick ML, Mouton CP, Oberman A, Perri MG, Sheps DS, Pettinger MB, Siscovick DS. Walking compared with vigorous exercise for the prevention of cardiovascular events in women. *N Engl J Med* 2002;347:716-725.
10.   Berlin JA, Colditz GA. A meta-analysis of physical activity in the prevention of coronary heart disease. *Am J Epidemiol* 1990;132:612-628.
11.   Taaffe DR. Sarcopenia—exercise as a treatment strategy. *Aust Fam Physician* 2006;35:130-134.
12.   Petersen AM, Pedersen BK. The anti-inflammatory effect of exercise. *J Appl Physiol* 2005;98:1154-1162.
13.   Rockhill B, Willett WC, Hunter DJ, Manson JE, Hankinson SE, Colditz GA. A prospective study of recreational physical activity and breast cancer risk. *Arch Intern Med* 1999;159:2290-2296.
14.   Giovannucci E, Ascherio A, Rimm EB, Colditz GA, Stampfer MJ, Willett WC. Physical activity, obesity, and risk for colon cancer and

adenoma in men. *Ann Intern Med* 1995;122:327-334.

15. Michaud DS, Giovannucci E, Willett WC, Colditz GA, Stampfer MJ, Fuchs CS. Physical activity, obesity, height, and the risk of pancreatic cancer. *JAMA* 2001;286:921-929.

16. Herbst RS, Bajorin DF, Bleiberg H, Blum D, Hao D, Johnson BE, Ozols RF, Demetri GD, Ganz PA, Kris MG, Levin B, Markman M, Raghavan D, Reaman GH, Sawaya R, Schuchter LM, Sweetenham JW, Vahdat LT, Vokes EE, Winn RJ, Mayer RJ. Clinical Cancer Advances 2005: Major Research Advances in Cancer Treatment, Prevention, and Screening—A Report From the American Society of Clinical Oncology. *J Clin Oncol* 2006;24:190-205.

17. Giovannucci EL, Liu Y, Leitzmann MF, Stampfer MJ, Willett WC. A prospective study of physical activity and incident and fatal prostate cancer. *Arch Intern Med* 2005;165:1005-1010.

18. Holmes MD, Chen WY, Feskanich D, Kroenke CH, Colditz GA.. Physical activity and survival after breast cancer diagnosis. *JAMA* 2005;293:2479-2486.

19. McNeely ML, Campbell KL, Rowe BH, Klassen TP, Mackey JR, Courneya KS. Effects of exercise on breast cancer patients and survivors: A systematic review and meta-analysis. *CMAJ* 2006;175:34-41.

20. Warburton DE, Nicol CW, Bredin SS. Health benefits of physical activity: The evidence. *CMAJ* 2006;174:801-809.

21. Malnick, S.D.H., Knobler, H. (2006). The medical complications of obesity. *QJM* 99: 565-579.

22. Calle EE, Rodriguez C, Walker-Thurmond K, Thun MJ. Overweight, obesity, and mortality from cancer in a prospectively studied cohort of U.S. adults. *N Engl J Med* 2003;348:1625-1638.

Chapter 13

1. Bossingham MJ, Carnell NS, Campbell WW. Water balance, hydration status, and fat-free mass hydration in younger and older adults. *Am J Clin Nutr* 2005;81:1342-1350.

2. Silva AM, Wang J, Pierson RN Jr, Wang Z, Heymsfield SB, Sardinha LB, Heshka S. Extracellular water: Greater expansion with age in African Americans. *J Appl Physiol* 2005;99:261-267.

3. Rothenbacher D, Low M, Hardt PD, Klor HU, Ziegler H, Brenner H. Prevalence and determinants of exocrine pancreatic insufficiency among older adults: Results of a population-based study. *Scand J Gastroenterol* 2005;40:697-704.

4. *Hydration and You*. The Beverage Institute for Health & Wellness. More information on the importance of hydration can be found at: http://www.beverageinstitute.com.

5. Sone Y, Kato N, Kojima Y, Takasu N, Tokura H. Effects of skin pressure by clothing on digestion and orocecal transit time of food. *J Physiol Anthropol Appl Human Sci* 2000;19:157-163.

6.   Humbert B, Nguyen P, Martin L, Dumon H, Vallette G, Maugere P, Darmaun D. Effect of glutamine on glutathione kinetics *in vivo* in dogs. *J Nutr Biochem* 2006; Mar 22.

7.   Topping DL, Clifton PM. Short-chain fatty acids and human colonic function: Roles of resistant starch and nonstarch polysaccharides. *Physiol Rev* 2001;81:1031-1064.

8.   Kay RM. Dietary fiber. *J Lipid Res* 1982;23:221-242.

9.   Dikeman CL, Murphy MR, Fahey GC Jr. Dietary fibers affect viscosity of solutions and simulated human gastric and small intestinal digesta. *J Nutr* 2006;136:913-919.

10. Institute of Medicine of the National Academies. Food and Nutrition Board. *Dietary Reference Intakes for Energy, Carbohydrate, Fiber, Fat, Fatty Acids, Cholesterol, Protein, and Amino Acids (Macronutrients), Chapter 7: Dietary, Functional, and Total Fiber.* The National Academies Press, Washington, D.C., 2005, pp. 339-421.

11. Michels KB, Fuchs CS, Giovannucci E, Colditz GA, Hunter DJ, Stampfer MJ, Willett WC. Fiber intake and incidence of colorectal cancer among 76,947 women and 47,279 men. *Cancer Epidemiol Biomarkers Prev* 2005;14:842-849.

12. Chandalia M, Garg A, Lutjohann D, von Bergmann K, Grundy SM, Brinkley LJ. Beneficial effects of high dietary fiber intake in patients with type 2 diabetes mellitus. *N Engl J Med* 2000;342:1392-1398.

13. He T, Priebe MG, Harmsen HJ, Stellaard F, Sun X, Welling GW, Vonk RJ.Colonic fermentation may play a role in lactose intolerance in humans. *J Nutr* 2006;136:58-63.

14. Nomoto K. Prevention of infections by probiotics. *J Biosci Bioeng* 2005;100:583-592.

15. Topping DL, Clifton PM. Short-chain fatty acids and human colonic function: Roles of resistant starch and nonstarch polysaccharides. *Physiol Rev* 2001;81:1031-1064.

16. Kay RM. Dietary fiber. *J Lipid Res* 1982;23:221-242.

17. Bouhnik Y, Raskine L, Simoneau G, Paineau D, Bornet F. The capacity of short-chain fructo-oligosaccharides to stimulate faecal bifidobacteria: A dose-response relationship study in healthy humans. *Nutr J* 2006;5:8 doi:10.1186/1475-2891-5-8 (http://www.nutritionj.com/content/5/1/8).

18. Tubelius P, Stan V, Zachrisson A. Increasing work-place healthiness with the probiotic *Lactobacillus reuteri*: A randomised, double-blind placebo-controlled study. *Environ Health* 2005;7;4:25 doi:10.1186/1476-069X-4-25 (http://www.ehjournal.net/content/4/1/25).

19. Rook GA, Brunet LR. Microbes, immunoregulation, and the gut. *Gut* 2005;54:317-320.

20. Shanahan F. Physiological basis for novel drug therapies used to treat the inflammatory bowel diseases. I. Pathophysiological basis and prospects for probiotic therapy in inflammatory bowel disease. *Am J Physiol Gastrointest Liver Physiol* 2005;288:G417-G421.

21. Chermesh I, Eliakim R. Probiotics and the gastrointestinal tract:

Where are we in 2005? *World J Gastroenterol* 2006;12:853-857.

22. Montalto M, Curigliano V, Santoro L, Vastola M, Cammarota G, Manna R, Gasbarrini A, Gasbarrini G. Management and treatment of lactose malabsorption. *World J Gastroenterol* 2006;12:187-191.

23. Hamilton-Miller JM. Probiotics and prebiotics in the elderly. *Postgrad Med J* 2004;80:447-451.

Chapter 14

1. Penninx BW, Kritchevsky SB, Newman AB, Nicklas BJ, Simonsick EM, Rubin S, Nevitt M, Visser M, Harris T, Pahor M. Inflammatory markers and incident mobility limitation in the elderly. *J Am Geriatr Soc* 2004;52:1105-1113.

2. Uribarri J, Cai W, Sandu O, Peppa M, Goldberg T, Vlassara H. Diet-derived advanced glycation end products are major contributors to the body's AGE pool and induce inflammation in healthy subjects. *Ann N Y Acad Sci* 2005;1043:461-466.

3. Couillard C, Pomerleau S, Ruel G, Archer WR, Bergeron J, Couture P, Lamarche B, Bergeron N. Associations between hypertriglyceridemia, dietary fat intake, oxidative stress, and endothelial activation in men. *Nutrition* 2006;22:600-608.

4. Colbert LH, Visser M, Simonsick EM, Tracy RP, Newman AB, Kritchevsky SB, Pahor M, Taaffe DR, Brach J, Rubin S, Harris TB. Physical activity, exercise, and inflammatory markers in older adults: Findings from the Health, Aging and Body Composition Study. *J Am Geriatr Soc* 2004;52:1098-1104.

5. Gao X, Bermudez OI, Tucker KL. Plasma C-reactive protein and homocysteine concentrations are related to frequent fruit and vegetable intake in Hispanic and non-Hispanic white elders. *J Nutr* 2004;134:913-918.

6. Li L, Sawamura T, Renier G. Glucose enhances human macrophage LOX-1 expression: Role for LOX-1 in glucose-induced macrophage foam cell formation. *Circ Res* 2004;94:892-901.

7. Sarkar D, Lebedeva IV, Emdad L, Kang DC, Baldwin AS Jr, Fisher PB. Human polynucleotide phosphorylase ($hPNPase^{old-35}$): A potential link between aging and inflammation. *Cancer Res* 2004;64:7473-7478.

8. Rosenblat M, Hayek T, Aviram M. Anti-oxidative effects of pomegranate juice (PJ) consumption by diabetic patients on serum and on macrophages. *Atherosclerosis* 2006;187:363-371.

9. Ferrucci L, Cherubini A, Bandinelli S, Bartali B, Corsi A, Lauretani F, Martin A, Andres-Lacueva C, Senin U, Guralnik JM. Relationship of plasma polyunsaturated fatty acids to circulating inflammatory markers. *J Clin Endocrinol Metab* 2006;91:439-446.

10. Ray AL, Semba RD, Walston J, Ferrucci L, Cappola AR, Ricks MO, Xue QL, Fried LP. Low serum selenium and total carotenoids predict mortality among older women living in the community: The Women's Health and Aging Studies. *J Nutr* 2006;136:172-176.

11. Schafer A, Chovanova Z, Muchova J, Sumegova K, Liptakova A, Durackova Z, Hogger P. Inhibition of COX-1 and COX-2 activity by plasma of human volunteers after ingestion of French maritime pine bark extract (Pycnogenol). *Biomed Pharmacother* 2006;60:5-9.
13. The Health Consequences of Smoking: A Report of the Surgeon General. [Atlanta, Ga.]: Dept. of Health and Human Services, Centers for Disease Control and Prevention, National Center for Chronic Disease Prevention and Health Promotion, Office on Smoking and Health; Washington, D.C., 2004 (available free at http://www.cdc.gov/tobacco/sgr/sgr_2004/index.htm).

Chapter 15

1. Gangwisch JE, Heymsfield SB, Boden-Albala B, Buijs RM, Kreier F, Pickering TG, Rundle AG, Zammit GK, Malaspina D. Short sleep duration as a risk factor for hypertension. Analyses of the first National Health and Nutrition Examination Survey. *Hypertension* 2006;47:833-839.
2. Ayas NT, White DP, Manson JE, Stampfer MJ, Speizer FE, Malhotra A, Hu FB. A prospective study of sleep duration and coronary heart disease in women. *Arch Intern Med* 2003;163:205-209.
3. Rajaratnam SM, Middleton B, Stone BM, Arendt J, Dijk DJ. Melatonin advances the circadian timing of EEG sleep and directly facilitates sleep without altering its duration in extended sleep opportunities in humans. *J Physiol* 2004;561:339-351.
4. Sofic E, Rimpapa Z, Kundurovic Z, Sapcanin A, Tahirovic I, Rustembegovic A, Cao G. Antioxidant capacity of the neurohormone melatonin. *J Neural Transm* 2005;112:349-358.
5. Burdakov D, Alexopoulos H. Metabolic state signalling through central hypocretin/orexin neurons. *J Cell Mol Med* 2005;9:795-803.
6. Markus CR, Jonkman LM, Lammers JH, Deutz NE, Messer MH, Rigtering N. Evening intake of -lactalbumin increases plasma tryptophan availability and improves morning alertness and brain measures of attention. *Am J Clin Nutr* 2005;81:1026-1033
7. Dietz BM, Mahady GB, Pauli GF, Farnsworth NR. Valerian extract and valerenic acid are partial agonists of the 5-HT$_{5a}$ receptor in vitro. *Mol Brain Res* 2005;138:191-197.
8. Goel N, Kim H, Lao RP. An olfactory stimulus modifies nighttime sleep in young men and women. *Chronobiol Int* 2005;22:889-904.
9. Goel N, Lao RP. Sleep changes vary by odor perception in young adults. *Biol Psychol* 2006;71:341-349.

Chapter 16

1. Giovannucci E, Rimm EB, Liu Y, Stampfer MJ, Willett WC. A prospective study of tomato products, lycopene, and prostate cancer risk. *J Natl Cancer Inst* 2002;94:391-398.
2. Etminan M, FitzGerald JM, Gleave M, Chambers K. Intake of

selenium in the prevention of prostate cancer: A systematic review and meta-analysis. *Cancer Causes Control* 2005;16:1125-1131.

3. Chun JY, Nadiminty N, Lee SO, Onate SA, Lou W, Gao AC. Mechanisms of selenium down-regulation of androgen receptor signaling in prostate cancer. *Mol Cancer Ther* 2006;5:913-918.

4. Sabichi AL, Lee JJ, Taylor RJ, Thompson IM, Miles BJ, Tangen CM, Minasian LM, Pisters LL, Caton JR, Basler JW, Lerner SP, Menter DG, Marshall JR, Crawford ED, Lippman SM. Selenium accumulation in prostate tissue during a randomized, controlled short-term trial of L-selenomethionine: A Southwest Oncology Group Study. *Clin Cancer Res* 2006;12:2178-2184.

5. Weinstein SJ, Wright ME, Pietinen P, King I, Tan C, Taylor PR, Virtamo J, Albanes D. Serum α-tocopherol and γ-tocopherol in relation to prostate cancer risk in a prospective study. *J Natl Cancer Inst* 2005;97:396-399.

6. Kirsh VA, Hayes RB, Mayne ST, Chatterjee N, Subar AF, Dixon LB, Albanes D, Andriole GL, Urban DA, Peters U; PLCO Trial. Supplemental and dietary vitamin E, beta-carotene, and vitamin C intakes and prostate cancer risk. *J Natl Cancer Inst* 2006;98:245-254.

7. Shiau CW, Huang JW, Wang DS, Weng JR, Yang CC, Lin CH, Li C, Chen CS. -Tocopheryl succinate induces apoptosis in prostate cancer cells in part through inhibition of Bcl-xL/Bcl-2 function. *J Biol Chem* 2006;281:11819-11825.

8. Limpens J, Schroder FH, de Ridder CM, Bolder CA, Wildhagen MF, Obermuller-Jevic UC, Kramer K, van Weerden WM. Combined lycopene and vitamin E treatment suppresses the growth of PC-346C human prostate cancer cells in nude mice. *J Nutr* 2006;136:1287-1293.

9. Mavi A, Terzi Z, Ozgen U, Yildirim A, Coskun M. Antioxidant properties of some medicinal plants: *Prangos ferulacea* (Apiaceae), *Sedum sempervivoides* (Crassulaceae), *Malva neglecta* (Malvaceae), *Cruciata taurica* (Rubiaceae), *Rosa pimpinellifolia* (Rosaceae), *Galium verum* subsp. *verum* (Rubiaceae), *Urtica dioica* (Urticaceae). *Biol Pharm Bull* 2004;27:702-705.

10. Safarinejad MR. *Urtica dioica* for treatment of benign prostatic hyperplasia. A prospective, randomized, double-blind, placebo-controlled, crossover study. *J Herb Pharmacother* 2005;5:1-11.

11. Wilt TJ, Ishani A, Stark G, MacDonald R, Lau J, Mulrow C. Saw palmetto extracts for treatment of benign prostatic hyperplasia. A systematic review. *JAMA* 1998;280:1604-1609.

12. Malik A, Mukhtar H. Prostate cancer prevention through pomegranate fruit. *Cell Cycle* 2006;5:371-373.

13. Malik A, Afaq F, Sarfaraz S, Adhami VM, Syed DN, Mukhtar H. Pomegranate fruit juice for chemoprevention and chemotherapy of prostate cancer. *Proc Natl Acad Sci U S A* 2005;102:14813-14818.

14. Ishani A, MacDonald R, Nelson D, Rutks I, Wilt TJ. *Pygeum africanum* for the treatment of patients with benign prostatic hyperplasia: A systematic review and quantitative meta-analysis. *Am J Med*

2000;109:654-664.

15. Wilt TJ, MacDonald R, Ishani A. beta-Sitosterol for the treatment
     of benign prostatic hyperplasia: A systematic review. *BJU Int*
     1999;83:976-983.

16. Kren V, Walterova D. Silybin and silymarin—new effects and
     applications. *Biomed Pap* 2005;149:29-41.

17. Costello LC, Franklin RB. The clinical relevance of the metabolism
     of prostate cancer; zinc and tumor suppression: Connecting the
     dots. *Mol Cancer* 2006;5:17 (13 pages). doi:10.1186/1476-4598-5-17
     (http://www.molecular-cancer.com/content/5/1/17).

18. Jones SB, DePrimo SE, Whitfield ML, Brooks JD. Resveratrol-induced
     gene expression profiles in human prostate cancer cells. *Cancer
     Epidemiol Biomarkers Prev* 2005;14:596-604.

19. John EM, Schwartz GG, Koo J, Van Den Berg D, Ingles SA. Sun
     exposure, vitamin D receptor gene polymorphisms, and risk of
     advanced prostate cancer. *Cancer Res* 2005;65:5470-5479.

20. Chan JM, Stampfer MJ, Ma J, Gann PH, Gaziano JM, Giovannucci EL.
     Dairy products, calcium, and prostate cancer risk in the Physicians'
     Health Study. *Am J Clin Nutr* 2001;74:549-554.

21. Baron JA, Beach M, Wallace K, Grau MV, Sandler RS, Mandel JS,
     Heber D, Greenberg ER. Risk of prostate cancer in a randomized
     clinical trial of calcium supplementation. *Cancer Epidemiol Biomarkers
     Prev* 2005;14:586-589.

22. Giovannucci E, Liu Y, Stampfer MJ, Willett WC. A prospective study
     of calcium intake and incident and fatal prostate cancer. *Cancer
     Epidemiol Biomarkers Prev* 2006;15:203-210.

23. Cross AJ, Peters U, Kirsh VA, Andriole GL, Reding D, Hayes RB, Sinha
     R. A prospective study of meat and meat mutagens and prostate
     cancer risk. *Cancer Res* 2005;65:11779-11784.

Chapter 17

1. Tarnopolsky MA. Mitochondrial DNA shifting in older adults following
    resistance exercise training. Appl Physiol Nutr Metab. 2009;34(3):348-54.

2. Abidoff M, Ramazanov Z. Rhodiola Rosea. The Herbal Heavyweight from
    Russia. National Bioscience Corp., Chester, NY, 2005, 6 pages.

3. De Bock K, Eijnde BO, Ramaekers M, Hespel P. Acute Rhodiola rosea intake
    can improve endurance exercise performance. Int J Sport Nutr Exerc Metab
    2004;14:298-307.

4. Ming DS, Hillhouse BJ, Guns ES, Eberding A, Xie S, Vimalanathan S,
    Towers GH. Bioactive compounds from Rhodiola rosea (Crassulaceae).
    Phytother Res 2005;19:740-743.

5. Mishra KP, Ganju L, Chanda S, Karan D, Sawhney RC. Aqueous extract of
    Rhodiola imbricata rhizome stimulates Toll-like receptor 4, granzyme-B and
    Th1 cytokines in vitro.Immunobiology. 2009;214(1):27-31.

6. Li HX, Sze SC, Tong Y, Ng TB. Production of Th1- and Th2-dependent
    cytokines induced by the Chinese medicine herb, Rhodiola algida, on human
    peripheral blood monocytes. J Ethnopharmacol. 2009;22;123(2):257-66.

Chapter 18

1. Abe K, Ijiri M, Suzuki T, Taguchi K, Koyama Y, Isemura M. Green tea with a high catechin content suppresses inflammatory cytokine expression in the galactosamine-injured rat liver. *Biomed Res* 2005;26:187-192.

2. Rana SV, Attri S, Vaiphei K, Pal R, Attri A, Singh K. Role of *N*-acetylcysteine in rifampicin-induced hepatic injury of young rats. *World J Gastroenterol* 2006;12:287-291.

3. Jonkers IJ, Smelt AH, Princen HM, Kuipers F, Romijn JA, Boverhof R, Masclee AA, Stellaard F. Fish oil increases bile acid synthesis in male patients with hypertriglyceridemia. *J Nutr* 2006;136:987-991.

4. He P, Court MH, Greenblatt DJ, von Moltke LL. Factors influencing midazolam hydroxylation activity in human liver microsomes. *Drug Metab Dispos* 2006;34:1198-1207.

5. Link LB, Potter JD. Raw versus cooked vegetables and cancer risk. *Cancer Epidemiol Biomarkers Prev* 2004;13:1422-1435.

6. *5 a Day – The Color Way.* Produce for Better Health Foundation. Wilmington, DE. http://www.5aday.org/html/colorway/colorway_home.php.

7. Lampe JW. Spicing up a vegetarian diet: Chemopreventive effects of phytochemicals. *Am J Clin Nutr* 2003;78(Suppl):579S-583S.

8. Harris WS, Sands SA, Windsor SL, Ali HA, Stevens TL, Magalski A, Porter CB, Borkon AM. Omega-3 fatty acids in cardiac biopsies from heart transplantation patients: Correlation with erythrocytes and response to supplementation. *Circulation* 2004;110:1645-1649.

9. Leitzmann MF, Willett WC, Rimm EB, Stampfer MJ, Spiegelman D, Colditz GA, Giovannucci E. A prospective study of coffee consumption and the risk of symptomatic gallstone disease in men. *JAMA* 1999;281:2106-2112.

10. Ruhl CE, Everhart JE. Association of coffee consumption with gallbladder disease. *Am J Epidemiol* 2000;152:1034-1038.

11. Tsai CJ, Leitzmann MF, Willett WC, Giovannucci EL. The effect of long-term intake of *cis* unsaturated fats on the risk for gallstone disease in men: A prospective cohort study. *Ann Intern Med* 2004;141:514-522.

12. Tsai CJ, Leitzmann MF, Willett WC, Giovannucci EL. Prospective study of abdominal adiposity and gallstone disease in US men. *Am J Clin Nutr* 2004;80:38-44.

13. Bilska A, Wlodek L. Lipoic acid — the drug of the future? *Pharmacol Rep* 2005;57:570-577.

14. Abe K, Ijiri M, Suzuki T, Taguchi K, Koyama Y, Isemura M. Green tea with a high catechin content suppresses inflammatory cytokine expression in the galactosamine-injured rat liver. *Biomed Res* 2005;26:187-192.

15. Zhang XH, Andreotti G, Gao YT, Deng J, Liu E, Rashid A, Wu K, Sun L, Sakoda LC, Cheng JR, Shen MC, Wang BS, Han TQ, Zhang BH, Gridley G, Fraumeni JF Jr, Hsing AW. Tea drinking and the risk of biliary tract cancers and biliary stones: A population-based case-control study in Shanghai, China. *Int J Cancer.* 2006;118:3089-3094.

16. Rana SV, Attri S, Vaiphei K, Pal R, Attri A, Singh K. Role of *N*-acetylcysteine

in rifampicin-induced hepatic injury of young rats. *World J Gastroenterol* 2006;12:287-291.

17. Jonkers IJ, Smelt AH, Princen HM, Kuipers F, Romijn JA, Boverhof R, Masclee AA, Stellaard F. Fish oil increases bile acid synthesis in male patients with hypertriglyceridemia. *J Nutr* 2006;136:987-991.

18. Farombi EO, Shrotriya S, Na HK, Kim SH, Surh YJ. Curcumin attenuates dimethylnitrosamine-induced liver injury in rats through Nrf2-mediated induction of heme oxygenase-1. *Food Chem Toxicol* 2008;46(4):1279-87.

19. Nishinaka T, Ichijo Y, Ito M, Kimura M, Katsuyama M, Iwata K, Miura T, Terada T, Yabe-Nishimura C. Curcumin activates human glutathione S-transferase P1 expression through antioxidant response element. *Toxicol Lett.* 2007;170(3):238-47.

Chapter 19

1. Wolf H, Grunwald M, Ecke GM, Zedlick D, Bettin S, Dannenberg C, Dietrich J, Eschrich K, Arendt T, Gertz HJ. The prognosis of mild cognitive impairment in the elderly. *J Neural Transm* 1998;54(Suppl.):31-50

2. Petersen RC, Smith GE, Waring SC, Ivnik RJ, Tangalos EG, Kokman E. Mild cognitive impairment: Clinical characterization and outcome. *Arch Neurol* 1999;56:303-308.

3. Johnson KA, Jones K, Holman BL. Preclinical prediction of Alzheimer's disease using SPECT. *Neurology* 1998;50:1563-1572.

4. Black SE. Can SPECT predict the future for mild cognitive impairment? *Can J Neurol Sci* 1999;26:4-6.

5. Ritchie K, Artero S, Touchon J. Classification criteria for mild cognitive impairment: a population-based validation study. *Neurology* 2001;56:37-42.

6. Tucker DM, Penland JG, Sandstead HH, Milne DB, Heck DG, Klevay LM. Nutrition status and brain function in aging. *Am J Clin Nutr* 1990;52:93-102.

7. McCaddon A. Homocysteine and cognitive impairment; a case series in a General Practice setting. *Nutr J* 2006; Feb 15;5:6. doi: 10.1186/1475-2891-5-6 (http://www.nutritionj.com/content/5/1/6).

8. Kalmijn S, Feskens EJM Launer LJ, Kromhout D. Polyunsaturated fatty acids, antioxidants, and cognitive function in very old men. *Am J Epidemiol* 1997;145:33-41.

9. Villardita C, Grioli S, Salmeri G. Nicoletti F, Pennisi G. Multicentre clinical trial of brain phosphatidylserine in elderly patients with intellectual deterioration. *Clin Trials J* 1987;24:84-93.

10. Palmieri G, Palmieri R, Inzoli MR, Lombardi G, Sottini C, Tavolato B, Giometto B. Double-blind controlled trial of phosphatidylserine in patients with senile mental deterioration. *Clin Trials J* 1987;24:73-83.

11. Crook T, Petrie W, Wells C, Massari DC. Effects of phosphatidylserine in Alzheimer's disease. *Psychopharmacol Bull* 1992;28:61-66.

12. Taylor CL. Letter regarding phosphatidylserine and cognitive dysfunction and dementia. US Food and Drug Administration.

13. Stough C, Clarke J, Lloyd J, Nathan PJ. Neuropsychological changes after 30-day Ginkgo biloba administration in healthy participants. Int J Neuropsychopharmacol 2001;4:131-134.

14. Subhan Z, Hindmarch I. The psychopharmacological effects of Ginkgo biloba extract in normal healthy volunteers. Int J Clin Pharmacol Res 1984;4:89-93.

15. Elsabagh S, Hartley DE, Ali O, Williamson EM, File SE. Differential cognitive effects of Ginkgo biloba after acute and chronic treatment in healthy young volunteers. Psychopharmacology (Berl). 2005;179(2):437-46.

16. Le Bars PL, Katz MM, Berman N, Itil TM, Freedman AM, Schatzberg AF. A placebo-controlled, double-blind, randomized trial of an extract of Ginkgo biloba for dementia. North American EGb Study Group. JAMA 1997;278(16):1327-32.

17. Institute of Medicine. Choline. In: Dietary Reference Intakes for Thiamin, Riboflavin, Niacin, Vitamin B_6, Folate, Vitamin B_{12}, Pantothenic Acid, Biotin and Choline. National Academy Press, Washington, DC, 1998, pp. 390-422.

18. Zaccheo O, Dinsdale D, Meacock PA, Glynn P. Neuropathy target esterase and its yeast homologue degrade phosphatidylcholine to glycerophosphocholine in living cells. J Biol Chem 2004;279:24024-24033.

19. Fernandez-Murray JP, McMaster CR. Glycerophosphocholine catabolism as a new route for choline formation for phosphatidylcholine synthesis by the Kennedy pathway. J Biol Chem 2005;280:38290-38296.

20. Amenta F, Tayebati SK, Vitali D, Di Tullio MA. Association with the cholinergic precursor choline alphoscerate and the cholinesterase inhibitor rivastigmine: An approach for enhancing cholinergic neurotransmission. Mech Ageing Dev 2006;127:173-179.

21. De Jesus Moreno Moreno M. Cognitive improvement in mild to moderate Alzheimer's dementia after treatment with the acetylcholine precursor choline alfoscerate: A multicenter, double-blind, randomized, placebo-controlled trial. Clin Ther 2003;25:178-193.

22. Parnetti L, Amenta F, Gallai V. Choline alfoscerate in cognitive decline and in acute cerebrovascular disease: An analysis of published clinical data. Mechs Aging Dev 2001;22:2041-2055.

23. Joseph JA, Shukitt-Hale B, Casadesus G. Reversing the deleterious effects of aging on neuronal communication and behavior: Beneficial properties of fruit polyphenolic compounds. Am J Clin Nutr 2005;81(Suppl.):313S-316S.

24. Coleston DM, Hindmarch I. Possible memory-enhancing properties of vinpocetine. Drug Develop Res 1988;14:191-193.

25. Subhan Z, Hindmarch I. Psychopharmacological effects of vinpocetine in normal healthy volunteers. Eur J Clin Pharmacol 1985;28:567-571.

26. Horvath B, Marton Z, Halmosi R, Alexy T, Szapary L, Vekasi J, Biro Z, Habon T, Kesmarky G, Toth K. In vitro antioxidant properties

of pentoxifylline, piracetam, and vinpocetine. *Clin Neuropharmacol* 2002;25(1):37-42.

27. Picconi B, Barone I, Pisani A, Nicolai R, Benatti P, Bernardi G, Calvani M, Calabresi P. Acetyl-L-carnitine protects striatal neurons against in vitro ischemia: The role of endogenous acetylcholine. *Neuropharmacology* 2006;50:917-923.

28. Passeri M, Iannuccelli M, Ciotti G, Bonati PA, Nolfe G, Cucinotta D. Mental impairment in aging: Selection of patients, methods of evaluation and therapeutic possibilities of acetyl-L-carnitine. *Int J Clin Pharmacol Res* 1988;8:367-376.

29. Passeri M, Cucinotta D, Bonati PA, Iannuccelli M, Parnetti L, Senin U. Acetyl-L-carnitine in the treatment of mildly demented elderly patients. *Int J Clin Pharmacol Res* 1990;10:75-79.

30. Montgomery SA, Thal LJ, Amrein R. Meta-analysis of double blind randomized controlled clinical trials of acetyl-L-carnitine versus placebo in the treatment of mild cognitive impairment and mild Alzheimer's disease. *Int Clin Psychopharmacol* 2003;18(2):61-71.

31. Ortega RM, Requejo AM, Lopez-Sobaler AM, Andres P, Navia B, Perea JM, Robles F. Cognitive function in elderly people is influenced by vitamin E status. *J Nutr* 2002;132:2065-2068.

32. Etminan M, Gill SS, Samii A. Intake of vitamin E, vitamin C, and carotenoids and the risk of Parkinson's disease: A meta-analysis. *Lancet Neurol* 2005;4:362-365.

33. Schweizer U, Brauer AU, Kohrle J, Nitsch R, Savaskan NE. Selenium and brain function: A poorly recognized liaison. *Brain Res Rev* 2004;45:164-178.

34. Chang RC, Chen W, Hudson P, Wilson B, Han DS, Hong JS. Neurons reduce glial responses to lipopolysaccharide (LPS) and prevent injury of microglial cells from over-activation by LPS. *J Neurochem* 2001;76:1042-1049.

35. Stella N, Estelles A, Siciliano J, Tence M, Desagher S, Piomelli D, Glowinski J, Premont J. Interleukin-1 enhances the ATP-evoked release of arachidonic acid from mouse astrocytes. *J Neurosci* 1997;17:2939-2946.

Chapter 20

1. Virtanen KA, Iozzo P, Hallsten K, Huupponen R, Parkkola R, Janatuinen T, Lonnqvist F, Viljanen T, Ronnemaa T, Lonnroth P, Knuuti J, Ferrannini E, Nuutila P. Increased fat mass compensates for insulin resistance in abdominal obesity and type 2 diabetes: A positron-emitting tomography study. *Diabetes* 2005;54:2720-2726.

2. Weickert MO, Mohlig M, Schofl C, Arafat AM, Otto B, Viehoff H, Koebnick C, Kohl A, Spranger J, Pfeiffer AF. Cereal fiber improves whole-body insulin sensitivity in overweight and obese women. *Diabetes Care* 2006;29:775-780.

3. Halton TL, Willett WC, Liu S, Manson JE, Stampfer MJ, Hu FB. Potato and French fry consumption and risk of type 2 diabetes in women.

Am J Clin Nutr 2006;83:284-290.

4. Schneeman BO. Qualified health claims: Letter of enforcement discretion — Chromium picolinate and insulin resistance (Docket No. 2004Q-0144) (letter). Office of Nutritional Products, Labeling, and Dietary Supplements, Center for Food Safety and Applied Nutrition, Food and Drug Administration, Washington, DC, August 25, 2005.

5. Lydic ML, McNurlan M, Bembo S, Mitchell L, Komaroff E, Gelato M. Chromium picolinate improves insulin sensitivity in obese subjects with polycystic ovary syndrome. *Fertil Steril* 2006;86:243-246.

6. Huerta MG, Roemmich JN, Kington ML, Bovbjerg VE, Weltman AL, Holmes VF, Patrie JT, Rogol AD, Nadler JL. Magnesium deficiency is associated with insulin resistance in obese children. *Diabetes Care* 2005;28:1175-1181.

7. Preet A, Gupta BL, Yadava PK, Baquer NZ. Efficacy of lower doses of vanadium in restoring altered glucose metabolism and antioxidant status in diabetic rat lenses. *J Biosci* 2005;30:221-230.

8. Kleefstra N, Houweling ST, Jansman FG, Groenier KH, Gans RO, Meyboom-de Jong B, Bakker SJ, Bilo HJ. Chromium treatment has no effect in patients with poorly controlled, insulin-treated type 2 diabetes in an obese Western population: A randomized, double-blind, placebo-controlled trial. *Diabetes Care* 2006;29:521-525.

9. Vanschoonbeek K, Thomassen BJ, Senden JM, Wodzig WK, van Loon LJ. Cinnamon supplementation does not improve glycemic control in postmenopausal type 2 diabetes patients. *J Nutr* 2006;136:977-980.

10. Ziegenfuss TN, Hofheins JE, Mendel RW, Landis J, Anderson RA. Effects of a water-soluble cinnamon extract on body composition and features of the metabolic syndrome in pre-diabetic men and women. *J Int Soc Sports Nutr* 2006;3:45-53.

11. Grassi D, Necozione S, Lippi C, Croce G, Valeri L, Pasqualetti P, Desideri G, Blumberg JB, Ferri C. Cocoa reduces blood pressure and insulin resistance and improves endothelium-dependent vasodilation in hypertensives. *Hypertension* 2005;46:398-405.

12. Gad MZ, El-Sawalhi MM, Ismail MF, El-Tanbouly ND. Biochemical study of the anti-diabetic action of the Egyptian plants Fenugreek and Balanites. *Mol Cell Biochem* 2006;281:173-183.

13. Anonymous. Gymnema sylvestre. *Altern Med Rev* 1999 Feb;4(1):46-7.

14. Preet A, Siddiqui MR, Taha A, Badhai J, Hussain ME, Yadava PK, Baquer NZ. Long-term effect of *Trigonella foenum graecum* and its combination with sodium orthovanadate in preventing histopathological and biochemical abnormalities in diabetic rat ocular tissues. *Mol Cell Biochem* 2006; May 23. doi: 10.1007/s11010-006-9156-0.

15. van Dam RM, Willett WC, Manson JE, Hu FB. Coffee, caffeine, and risk of type 2 diabetes: A prospective cohort study in younger and middle-aged U.S. women. *Diabetes Care* 2006;29:398-403.

16. Pereira MA, Parker ED, Folsom AR. Coffee consumption and risk of

type 2 diabetes mellitus. *Arch Intern Med* 2006;166:1311-1316.

17. van Dijk AE, Olthof MR, Meeuse JC, Seebus E, Heine RJ, van Dam
     RM. Acute effects of decaffeinated coffee and the major coffee
     components chlorogenic acid and trigonelline on glucose tolerance.
     Diabetes Care 2009;32(6):1023-5.

Chapter 21

1. Ottillinger B, Greeske K. Rational therapy of chronic venous
    insufficiency—chances and limits of the therapeutic use of
    horse-chestnut seeds extract. *BMC Cardiovasc Disord* 2001;1:5.
    doi:10.1186/1471-2261-1-5 (http://www.biomedcentral.com/1471-
    2261/1/5).
2. Sato I, Kofujita H, Suzuki T, Kobayashi H, Tsuda S. Antiinflammatory
    effect of Japanese horse chestnut (*Aesculus turbinata*) seeds. *J Vet Med
    Sci* 2006;68:487-489.
3. Pittler MH, Ernst E. Horse chestnut seed extract for chronic venous
    insufficiency. *Cochrane Database Syst Rev* 2006;(1):CD003230.
4. Ramelet AA. Daflon 500 mg: Symptoms and edema. Clinical update.
    Angiology 2005;56 (Suppl.):S25-S32.
5. Smith PC. Daflon 500 mg and venous leg ulcer: New results from a
    meta-analysis. *Angiology* 2005;56 (Suppl.):S33-S39.

Chapter 22

1. Age-Related Eye Disease Study Research Group. A randomized,
    placebo-controlled, clinical trial of high-dose supplementation with
    vitamins C and E, beta carotene, and zinc for age-related macular
    degeneration and vision loss. *Arch Opthalmol* 2001;119:1417-1436.
2. Beatty S, Boulton M, Henson D, Koh H-H, Murray IJ. Macular
    pigment and age related macular degeneration. *Br J Ophthalmol*
    1999;83:867–877.
3. Beatty S, Murray IJ, Henson DB, Carden D, Koh H-H, Boulton ME.
    Macular pigment and risk for age-related macular degeneration in
    subjects from a Northern European population. *Invest Ophthalmol Vis
    Sci* 2001;42:439-446.
4. Richer S, Stiles W, Statkute L, Pulido J, Frankowski J, Rudy D, Pei
    K, Tsipursky M, Nyland J. Double-masked, placebo-controlled,
    randomized trial of lutein and antioxidant supplementation in
    the intervention of atrophic age-related macular degeneration: The
    Veterans LAST study (Lutein Antioxidant Supplementation Trial).
    Optometry 2004;75:216-230.
5. Seddon JM, Ajani UA, Sperduto RD, Hiller R, Blair N, Burton TC,
    Farber MD, Gragoudas ES, Haller J, Miller DT, *et al.* (1994) Dietary
    carotenoids, vitamins A, C, and E, and advanced age-related macular
    degeneration. Eye Disease Case-Control Study Group. *JAMA*
    1994;272:1413-1420.
6. Jacques PF, Chylack LT Jr, Hankinson SE, Khu PM, Rogers G, Friend

J, Tung W, Wolfe JK, Padhye N, Willett WC, Taylor A. Long-term nutrient intake and early age-related nuclear lens opacities. *Arch Ophthalmol* 2001;119:1009-1019.

7. Unlu NZ, Bohn T, Clinton SK, Schwartz SJ. Carotenoid absorption from salad and salsa by humans is enhanced by the addition of avocado or avocado oil. *J Nutr* 2005;135:431-436.

8. Burke JD, Curran-Celentano J, Wenzel AJ. Diet and serum carotenoid concentrations affect macular pigment optical density in adults 45 years and older. *J Nutr* 2005;135:1208-1214.

9. Rodriguez-Carmona M, Kvansakul J, Harlow JA, Kopcke W, Schalch W, Barbur JL. The effects of supplementation with lutein and/or zeaxanthin on human macular pigment density and colour vision. *Ophthalmic Physiol Opt* 2006;26:137-147.

10. Dene BA, Maritim AC, Sanders RA, Watkins JB 3rd. Effects of antioxidant treatment on normal and diabetic rat retinal enzyme activities. *J Ocul Pharmacol Ther* 2005;21:28-35.

11. Aragona P, Papa V, Micali A, Santocono M, Milazzo G. Long term treatment with sodium hyaluronate-containing artificial tears reduces ocular surface damage in patients with dry eye. *Br J Ophthalmol* 2002;86:181-184.

12. Debbasch C, De La Salle SB, Brignole F, Rat P, Warnet JM, Baudouin C. Cytoprotective effects of hyaluronic acid and Carbomer 934P in ocular surface epithelial cells. *Invest Ophthalmol Vis Sci* 2002;43:3409-3415.

Chapter 23

1. Gulati OP. Pycnogenol® in venous disorders: A review. *Eur Bull Drug Res* 1999;7:8-13.

2. Belcaro G, Cesarone MR, Errichi BM, Ledda A, Di Renzo A, Stuard S, Dugall M, Pellegrini L, Rohdewald P, Ippolito E, Ricci A, Cacchio M, Ruffini I, Fano F, Hosoi M. Venous ulcers: Microcirculatory improvement and faster healing with local use of Pycnogenol. *Angiology* 2005;56:699-705.

3. Cesarone MR, Belcaro G, Rohdewald P, Pellegrini L, Ledda A, Vinciguerra G, Ricci A, Gizzi G, Ippolito E, Fano F, Dugall M, Acerbi G, Cacchio M, Di Renzo A, Hosoi M, Stuard S, Corsi M. Comparison of Pycnogenol and Daflon in treating chronic venous insufficiency: A prospective, controlled study. *Clin Appl Thromb Hemost* 2006;12:205-212.

4. Trommer H, Neubert RH. Screening for new antioxidative compounds for topical administration using skin lipid model systems. *J Pharm Pharm Sci* 2005;8:494-506.

5. Yoshimura M, Watanabe Y, Kasai K, Yamakoshi J, Koga T. Inhibitory effect of an ellagic acid-rich pomegranate extract on tyrosinase activity and ultraviolet-induced pigmentation. *Biosci Biotechnol Biochem* 2005;69:2368-2373.

6. Syed DN, Malik A, Hadi N, Sarfaraz S, Afaq F, Mukhtar H.

Photochemopreventive effect of pomegranate fruit extract on UVA-mediated activation of cellular pathways in normal human epidermal keratinocytes. *Photochem Photobiol* 2006;82:398-405.

7. Song XZ, Bi ZG, Xu AE. Green tea polyphenol epigallocatechin-3-gallate inhibits the expression of nitric oxide synthase and generation of nitric oxide induced by ultraviolet B in HaCaT cells. *Chin Med J* 2006;119:282-287.

8. Heinrich U, Neukam K, Tronnier H, Sies H, Stahl W. Long-term ingestion of high flavanol cocoa provides photoprotection against UV-induced erythema and improves skin condition in women. *J Nutr* 2006;136:1565-1569.

9. Boelsma E, van de Vijver LP, Goldbohm RA, Klopping-Ketelaars IA, Hendriks HF, Roza L. Human skin condition and its associations with nutrient concentrations in serum and diet. *Am J Clin Nutr* 2003;77:348-355.

Chapter 24

1. International Osteoporosis Foundation. Osteoporosis: Teaching Slide Kit. Lyon, France. (http://www.osteofound.org/health_professionals/teaching_resources/slide_kit.html)

2. Reid IR, Ames RW, Evans MC, Gamble GD, Sharpe SJ. Long-term effects of calcium supplementation on bone loss and fractures in postmenopausal women: A randomized controlled trial. *Am J Med* 1995;98:331-335.

3. Recker RR, Hinders S, Davies KM, Heaney RP, Stegman MR, Lappe JM, Kimmel DB. Correcting calcium nutritional deficiency prevents spine fractures in elderly women. *J Bone Miner Res* 1996;11:1961-1966.

4. Riggs BL, Seeman E, Hodgson SF, Taves DR, O'Fallon WM. Effect of the fluoride/calcium regimen on vertebral fracture occurrence in postmenopausal osteoporosis. Comparison with conventional therapy. *N Engl J Med* 1982;306:446-450.

5. Bischoff-Ferrari HA, Willett WC, Wong JB, Giovannucci E, Dietrich T, Dawson-Hughes B. Fracture prevention with vitamin D supplementation: A meta-analysis of randomized controlled trials. *JAMA* 2005;293:2257-2264.

6. Jackson RD, LaCroix AZ, Gass M, Wallace RB, Robbins J, Lewis CE, Bassford T, Beresford SA, Black HR, Blanchette P, Bonds DE, Brunner RL, Brzyski RG, Caan B, Cauley JA, Chlebowski RT, Cummings SR, Granek I, Hays J, Heiss G, Hendrix SL, Howard BV, Hsia J, Hubbell FA, Johnson KC, Judd H, Kotchen JM, Kuller LH, Langer RD, Lasser NL, Limacher MC, Ludlam S, Manson JE, Margolis KL, McGowan J, Ockene JK, O'Sullivan MJ, Phillips L, Prentice RL, Sarto GE, Stefanick ML, Van Horn L, Wactawski-Wende J, Whitlock E, Anderson GL, Assaf AR, Barad D; Women's Health Initiative Investigators. Calcium plus vitamin D supplementation and the risk of fractures. *N Engl J Med* 2006;354:669-683.

7. Porthouse J, Cockayne S, King C, Saxon L, Steele E, Aspray T, Baverstock M, Birks Y, Dumville J, Francis R, Iglesias C, Puffer S, Sutcliffe A, Watt I, Torgerson DJ. Randomised controlled trial of calcium and supplementation with cholecalciferol (vitamin D3) for prevention of fractures in primary care. *BMJ* 2005;330:1003 (6 pages). doi:10.1136/bmj.330.7498.1003 (http://bmj.com/cgi/content/full/330/7498/1003).

8. DeLuca HF. Overview of general physiologic features and functions of vitamin D. *Am J Clin Nutr* 2004;80(Suppl.):1689S-1696S.

9. Macdonald HM, New SA, Golden MH, Campbell MK, Reid DM. Nutritional associations with bone loss during the menopausal transition: Evidence of a beneficial effect of calcium, alcohol, and fruit and vegetable nutrients and of a detrimental effect of fatty acids. *Am J Clin Nutr* 2004;79:155-165.

10. Maggio D, Barabani M, Pierandrei M, Polidori MC, Catani M, Mecocci P, Senin U, Pacifici R, Cherubini A. Marked decrease in plasma antioxidants in aged osteoporotic women: Results of a cross-sectional study. *J Clin Endocrinol Metab* 2003;88:1523-7152.

11. Ryder KM, Shorr RI, Bush AJ, Kritchevsky SB, Harris T, Stone K, Cauley J, Tylavsky FA. Magnesium intake from food and supplements is associated with bone mineral density in healthy older white subjects.J Am Geriatr Soc. 2005 Nov;53(11):1875-80.

12. Nielsen FH, Hunt CD, Mullen LM, Hunt JR. Effect of dietary boron on mineral, estrogen, and testosterone metabolism in postmenopausal women. *FASEB J* 1987;1:394-397.

13. Weiss LA, Barrett-Connor E, von Muhlen D. Ratio of n-6 to n-3 fatty acids and bone mineral density in older adults: The Rancho Bernardo Study. *Am J Clin Nutr* 2005;81:934-938.

14. Corwin RL, Hartman TJ, Maczuga SA, Graubard BI. Dietary saturated fat intake is inversely associated with bone density in humans: Analysis of NHANES III. *J Nutr* 2006;136:159-165.

15. Dawson-Hughes B, Harris SS, Rasmussen H, Song L, Dallal GE. Effect of dietary protein supplements on calcium excretion in healthy older men and women. *J Clin Endocrinol Metab* 2004;89:1169-1173.

16. Przkora R, Herndon DN, Suman OE, Jeschke MG, Meyer WJ, Chinkes DL, Mlcak RP, Huang T, Barrow RE. Beneficial effects of extended growth hormone treatment after hospital discharge in pediatric burn patients. *Ann Surg* 2006;243:796-801.

17. Potter SM, Baum JA, Teng H, Stillman RJ, Shay NF, Erdman JW Jr. Soy protein and isoflavones: Their effects on blood lipids and bone density in postmenopausal women. *Am J Clin Nutr* 1998;68(Suppl.):1375S-1379S.

18. Alekel DL, Germain AS, Peterson CT, Hanson KB, Stewart JW, Toda T. Isoflavone-rich soy protein isolate attenuates bone loss in the lumbar spine of perimenopausal women. *Am J Clin Nutr* 2000;72:844-852.

19. Roughead ZK, Hunt JR, Johnson LK, Badger TM, Lykken GI. Controlled substitution of soy protein for meat protein: Effects on calcium retention, bone, and cardiovascular health indices in

postmenopausal women. *J Clin Endocrinol Metab* 2005;90:181-189.

20. Arjmandi BH, Lucas EA, Khalil DA, Devareddy L, Smith BJ, McDonald J, Arquitt AB, Payton ME, Mason C. One year soy protein supplementation has positive effects on bone formation markers but not bone density in postmenopausal women. *Nutr J* 2005;4:8. doi:10.1186/1475-2891-4-8 (http://www.nutritionj.com/content/4/1/8).

21. Gennari C, Agnusdei D, Crepaldi G, Isaia G, Mazzuoli G, Ortolani S, Bufalino L, Passeri M. Effect of ipriflavone—a synthetic derivative of natural isoflavones—on bone mass loss in the early years after menopause. *Menopause* 1998;5:9-15.

22. Alexandersen P, Toussaint A, Christiansen C, Devogelaer JP, Roux C, Fechtenbaum J, Gennari C, Reginster JY; Ipriflavone Multicenter European Fracture Study. Ipriflavone in the treatment of postmenopausal osteoporosis: A randomized controlled trial. *JAMA* 2001;285:1482-1488.

23. Cockayne S, Adamson J, Lanham-New S, Shearer MJ, Gilbody S, Torgerson DJ. Vitamin K and the prevention of fractures: Systematic review and meta-analysis of randomized controlled trials. *Arch Intern Med* 2006;166:1256-1261.

24. Celestini M, Marchese A, Serenelli A, Graziani G. A randomized controlled trial on the efficacy of physical exercise in patients braced for instability of the lumbar spine. *Eura Medicophys* 2005;41:223-231.

25. Chakkalakal DA. Alcohol-induced bone loss and deficient bone repair. *Alcohol Clin Exp Res* 2005;29:2077-2090.

26. Kaukonen JP, Nurmi-Luthje I, Luthje P, Naboulsi H, Tanninen S, Kataja M, Kallio ML, Leppilampi M. Acute alcohol use among patients with acute hip fractures: A descriptive incidence study in southeastern Finland. *Alcohol Alcohol* 2006;41:345-348.

Chapter 25

1. Scott JE, Stockwell RA. Cartilage elasticity resides in shape module decoran and aggrecan sumps of damping fluid. Implications in osteoarthrosis. *J Physiol* 2006; Mar. 31. doi: 10.1113/jphysiol.2006.108100 (http://jp.physoc.org/cgi/content/abstract/jphysiol.2006.108100v1).

2. Herbert AA, Kondo CR, Almendra CL, Matsuo T, Dichi I. Supplementation of fish oil and olive oil in patients with rheumatoid arthritis. *Nutrition* 2005;21:131-136.

3. Goldberg RJ, Katz J. A meta-analysis of the analgesic effects of omega-3 polyunsaturated fatty acid supplementation for inflammatory joint pain. *Pain* 2007;129(1-2):210-23.

4. Flex Protex 197 Drovanti A, Bignamini AA, Rovati AL. Therapeutic activity of oral glucosamine sulfate in osteoarthrosis: A placebo-controlled double-blind investigation. *Clin Ther* 1980;3:260-272.

5. Flex Protex 198 Rovati LC. Clinical research in osteoarthritis: Design and results of shot-term and long-term trials with disease-modifying